A Playful Approach to Restoration Therapy

This accessible guide provides family and play therapists with an innovative method for addressing maladaptive emotional behavior in vulnerable children, helping them develop a practical understanding of how to diagnose, treat, and help children move from pain to peace.

Drawing from Frigaard's years of experience, this book presents the scientific model behind restoration play therapy and anticipates the multiple directions that healing and recovery might take. This guide combines creative and directive approaches to collaborative play with the vision to create deep-rooted change in clients. Including step-by-step session plans as well as introducing metaphorical "coping characters," Brutus the Blaming Badger, Sharla the Shameful Sheep, Contessa the Controlling Cow and Eddie the Escape Goat, the chapters encourage a therapeutic play environment that draws upon accessible techniques, empowering children to regain control of their responses to emotional pain. By moving between a framework of practical insight and its creative application, this text ensures therapists engage with clients where they are and build empathetic relationships with them.

This book is invaluable reading for family and play therapists as well as other mental health professionals that work with children. The book encourages parents and educators to be part of the healing process, and they can also use the techniques with the children in their lives.

Nancy Frigaard, D.Min., is a Licensed Marriage and Family Therapist, educator and clinical supervisor. She has worked as a faculty member at Fuller Theological Seminary and an adjunct faculty member at Arizona Christian University. She is currently occupied as Director of Fuller Seminary Arizona, Marriage and Family Therapy Program. She is also an assistant professor. Her private practice specializes in working with children, adolescents, parents, families, foster care, and adoption issues.

What do you think of when you think of the word "play?" Creativity? Engagement? Imagination? Maybe even words like growth and development come to mind. In her brilliant work of applying restoration therapy to a play setting, Nancy Frigaard extends our understanding of how attachment, emotional regulation and mindfulness can be skillfully engaged in the work with children. As important, you will quickly see how this playful approach helps families by changing the lives of children. Not only does her approach chart a course for potential and change in therapy, the result is perfectly suited for play therapy: It is fun!

Terry D. Hargrave, Ph.D., *Evelyn and Frank Freed Professor of Marriage and Family Therapy, Fuller Theological Seminary*

A Playful Approach to Restoration Therapy: Helping Kids Play Their Way From Pain to Peace is a very worthwhile resource not just for professional counselors but for the church and any type of ministry for children.

Dr. H. Norman Wright, *DMIN., MFCC, CTS, Author of over ninety books*

A Playful Approach to Restoration Therapy

Helping Kids Play their Way
from Pain to Peace

Nancy Frigaard

Routledge
Taylor & Francis Group

NEW YORK AND LONDON

Cover image: Getty Images

First published 2023
by Routledge
605 Third Avenue, New York, NY 10158

and by Routledge
4 Park Square, Milton Park, Abingdon, Oxon, OX14 4RN

Routledge is an imprint of the Taylor & Francis Group, an informa business

© 2023 Nancy Frigaard

Library of Congress Cataloging-in-Publication Data
A catalog record for this book has been requested

ISBN: 978-0-367-45811-9 (hbk)
ISBN: 978-0-367-45813-3 (pbk)
ISBN: 978-1-003-02550-4 (ebk)

DOI: 10.4324/9781003025504

Typeset in Bembo
by Apex CoVantage, LLC

This work is nonfiction, although many of the names and personal characteristics have been changed in order to disguise their identities. Any resemblance to any individual living or dead is completely coincidental and unintentional.

For my parents Roxy and John Clum—my life-long lifelines.

Mom, you are my greatest mentor, teacher and friend. You are the smartest person I know. If someone in the family deserves a doctorate for years of relentless research and study it is you, not I.

Dad, your life example has taught me that the fruit of vision will not bear without rolling up sleeves and getting to work. It is no wonder you grow the grandest, greenest, gardens in the Great Northwest.

I deeply admire and long to emulate your example of fearless expenditures of energy on hard work and joy-filled service to others.

Contents

Acknowledgments

To Dr. Terry D. Hargrave, Dr. H. Norman Wright, Dr. Kimberly Bailey, and Dr. Debra Merrifield What a privilege it has been to sit at your feet and glean from your years of hard work in the counseling field. Each of you is great and humble at once, not seeking power over others but to empower them. Thank you for teaching me this lesson well. I intend to honor it by passing this blessing on to those whom I am privileged to lead, train, supervise and counsel.

To my husband, Rick. I appreciate you, your love and desire to grow together. I am filled with thankfulness when I recall the long hours and time you provided me to complete this project. Your overall character of helpfulness when anyone is in need is something I have long admired.

To my children, Michele and Micah:

Michele, you embody the two pillars of a healthy relationship that this book speaks of: love and trustworthiness. Your integrity is sure and lived through a lens of love. I am ecstatic to welcome you into the field of Marriage and Family Therapy.

Micah, despite all of the time I have spent with you, your creative talents still astonish me. Thank you for sharing your skills to help complete this work. Your joy and love for children are infectious. I am deeply proud of you.

Preface and Introduction

Preface

Play therapy has been almost entirely non-directive in its approach until now. Although this is effective at times, non-directive play can leave both the therapist and client in an ambiguous state, feeling unsure of their work and progress. Restoration Therapy: helping kids play their way from pain to peace is an innovative approach that is both directive and experiential in nature. The approach allows pediatric clients to work within a framework of choices that make sound clinical sense. It provides both new and seasoned therapists with a clear picture of how to move forward in their work with children. The therapist can observe therapeutic goals being met in measurable ways while learning to work within a structure that leaves much room for creative play.

Therapy has long been touted as an art and a science. The subtle nuances and creative art of client care, including things like adaptive attunement, warmth, compassion, and novelty, are non-negotiable. Without these characteristics, the counseling room becomes stale, clinical, cold, and ineffective. Children need to be able to play creatively, express freely, and experience compassion and warmth.

Equally important is the child's need to be guided by informed therapists who are well versed in the science of counseling. Clinicians need to be well informed of how the brain responds to emotional pain and the reactive behaviors that will inevitably ensue. Restoration Therapy is a scientifically informed approach with proven structure and sequence that works to calm the upset, emotional midbrain. This allows the child to experience physiological, cognitive, and emotional relief.

Restoration Play Therapy is a unique blend of the art and science of therapy for children. It prepares counselors with a practical understanding of how to diagnose, treat, and help children move from pain to peace. The narrative provides the therapist with valuable insights and specific tools to orchestrate a thriving therapeutic play environment. In this milieu filled with love and safety, the client learns to experience peace while practicing new and effective behaviors. These interventions create deeply rooted change in the form of newly built neurological pathways. Restoration Play Therapy is creative and directive in scope auguring greater success and peace for both the pediatric therapist and client.

As the field of Restoration Therapists continues to grow, observable positive patient outcomes are undeniable. Questions regarding how to apply this theory to children are quickly on the rise. Restoration Play Therapy: helping kids play their way from pain to peace is meant to answer theoretical application's pragmatic questions.

Through both a directive and experiential approach, the clinician walks children through an experience of moving from emotional pain to peace. Many adult clients have already discovered emotional healing and relief through the implementation of restoration therapy. This book allows children an opportunity to experience the same in their own language of play.

The work is creatively scripted and illustrated with metaphorical characters equipping the therapist with innovative material aiding pediatric patient progress. For example, the clinician joins the child in discovering how they are dealing with their emotional pain through maladaptive behaviors. The four main "coping characters" that appear are Brutus the Blaming Badger, Shilo the Shameful Sheep, Contessa the Controlling Cow, and Eddie the Escape Goat. Through the use of these captivating characters, along with others, the reader gains methodology for guided collaborative play with the client.

Restoration Play Therapy: helping kids play their way from pain to peace is written with a tenor of compassion for the observed powerlessness that children often feel when faced with interpersonal or intrapersonal conflict. The painful primary ensuing emotions of feeling unsafe or unloved can be overwhelming to manage alone. This book arms the therapist to equip and empower children who are some of the most vulnerable and powerless among us.

Introduction

As a previous student of Marital and Family Therapy and as a current instructor of Family Studies in the university setting, I have observed that there is a barren place in the field of marriage and family therapy. There is little to no teaching regarding individual work with children. There is a pressing need to bring direction and relief to both clinicians and pediatric clients who find themselves in situations where parents are unable or unwilling to be a part of their child's therapeutic journey.

Strangely, there appear to be forms of subtle and sometimes overt cynicism and or ageism regarding the efficacy of working with kids apart from their family system's physical presence. True to the form of a licensed marriage and family therapist, I agree that if we can work directly with the child's family system in part or its entirety, it garners undeniable positive outcomes (Kaslow, 1996). However, there are many times that this is simply not possible. When it is impossible to work directly with parents or primary caregivers, we find ourselves face-to-face with a child apart from his system. What is a marriage and family therapist to do in these circumstances?

Just as with adults, we still conceptualize the patient within a socio-ecological framework and work with them accordingly. We press on toward helping this hurting human before us, male or female, big or small, pre- or post-pubescent; our job is to help them find freedom from their pain and emotional healing. More specifically, as marriage and family therapists, we endeavor to continue to work to create change within their system to usher in healing for both them and their families. For whatever reasons, the efficacy of children leading in system change has been largely unexplored; the idea is crucified on the ideal top-down approach's altar.

As with most of our clients, we often have to adapt our work when the ideal is unattainable. For instance, when a spouse refuses to attend the session, we march forward, believing if the present individual can change, the system will follow suit. We sound significantly less hopeful when faced with individual work with children. I have heard following sentiments from respected people in the field of marriage and family therapy describe some of the negative beliefs regarding pediatric practice:

> "I put in my time with kids as a new therapist and thank God that I have graduated from working with them."
>
> "I only allow my new interns to see kids in case they make a mistake."
>
> "Kids exhaust me."
>
> "I don't work with children; they just go back into their family system and get ruined all over again. It feels like an effort in futility."
>
> "Kids can't really change unless we work with the parents. I refuse to see children If their parents won't come with them to the session."
>
> "In family systems work, we need to use a 'top-down' approach. It puts too much pressure on a child to expect them to change first."

While parts of the quotes above may be genuine, in their entirety, they are false. Even Restoration Therapy holds to a belief that parents are the original brain programmers. While this is true, it does not mean that reprogramming or programming anew is impossible. I hope to challenge these unhelpful beliefs held by most in the field of marriage and family therapy. Weeds grow in every good field. This idea that we cannot adequately help children individually is nothing less than a weed. It is time it is plucked at the root so that greater health for kids and their families can start growing in its place. There is nothing more beautiful than the minds and souls of children. This book will help to till the hardened ground of unexplored territory and ready the soil for new growth and subsequent beauty.

Many clinicians appear stuck singing these memorized, futile-sounding songs, quoting mantras contrary to our core beliefs of being helpful and hopeful. Early on, I was guilty of similar statements. I was scared to see children individually and felt ill-equipped. I, too, clung to the belief that this family system work was primarily for adults or families who presented together in session. I felt guilty for taking money for a session with a child whose parents refused to come. I was earning a significantly higher rate than the average babysitter, and my ethics were bothered by this because I wasn't sure I could do much good. I believed what I had been taught.

It is part of our nature to trend toward believing what we are taught. It is impossible to think in deeply critical ways about every teaching we hear, each dissonant note or inappropriate lyric that crosses our path. We often merely "sing-along" without exploring its meaning or listening to see if it genuinely is congruent with our values. We go on repeating and passing on lyrics that may not beneficial or even the slightest bit accurate.

This tendency is reminiscent of a story a dear friend from Texas relayed to me. She and her six-year-old daughter were riding in the car on their way to church. My friend turned up the radio as she noticed her daughter singing robustly along with Dolly Parton and Kenny Rogers to the song *Islands in The Stream*. Toward the end of the chorus, there is a line that refers to the couple's reliance on the other. She heard her six-year-old clearly sing the following lyrics: "and they *will lie upon each* other ah-ah." My friend turned down the radio, incredulous that her daughter was so boldly singing these inappropriate lines. After being frantically corrected by her mother for this lurid-sounding rendition of the song, the six-year-old maintained that these were indeed the words and she had done nothing wrong. She argued that she had heard her Mom sing the same thing to her one-hundred times, and she was not very nice to get mad at her for it! My friend chuckled, and her frustration melted into laughter.

Like my friend's daughter, we have all sung along with lyrics that we have yet to think through or validate critically. In so doing, we likely have come across as inappropriate or obtuse, when in reality, our words are an innocent reflection of what we have heard and understood to be accurate.

The quotes mentioned above have come from Marriage and Family therapists and instructors for whom I have the highest respect. After I began working with children, each time I witnessed these proclamations, there was a part of me that saw their point. I agreed and disagreed at once. This, in turn, provoked a myriad of uneasy feelings within me. I am currently teaching a General Psychology course at the university where I work. The textbook asserts, "the three foundational components of critical scientific thinking within the world of psychology are curiosity, skepticism and humility" (Myers & DeWall, 2010).

These three components described my "uneasiness" perfectly when I heard the statements about working with children. My curiosity sprung to life because I wondered how children were to be helped under the umbrella of family systems if their parents refused to participate in the session or, God forbid, outside of the session. I am a proponent of Salvador Minuchin and Structural Therapy. I whole-heartedly concede that the top-down approach is ideal (Minuchin & Fishman, 1998). I agree that parents are responsible for doing their own work, and as they become healthy, the child will follow suit. I concur that parents are the original brain programmers and are endowed with significant power to lead their children into flourishing or languishing places. I preach the power of parenting in my classrooms and therapeutic sessions.

When I read the biblical account of Jesus making known to humankind their purpose of "going and making disciples" (Matt. 28:19, NIV), I often take this quite literally, knowing that when we procreate, we make disciples. The word disciple simply means "follower." Whether for good or bad, our kids are our disciples.

This concept of parents having power in the lives of their children is inarguable. I think parental influence is so evident that this is part of why the field has held unwaveringly to this ideal. If we were living in a world where things are as they should be, a world where parents took this job seriously and were healthy enough to create healthy followers, we could remain with tightly gripped hands still holding fast to this idea that parents must be the ones to induce change. They must first do the work to receive insight and then embrace the arduous task of experiential change. I think it is correct and appropriate to explore and even root for this type of order as we work for system change. Historically, renowned therapists have refused to work with any individual in the system, including children, but required the entire family to come to the session. Carl Whitaker recounts times when he would send the family home or wait together an uncomfortable amount of time to begin the session until all had arrived (Napier &Whitaker, 1978). This is an okay approach to have; however, as families become more fragmented, the more complicated it is to see them together.

Problems arise when parents, for various reasons, are absent or refusing to do any sort of work for their children to bring them into a place of emotional health. *Do we wipe our hands clean of the matter perpetuating a system of adult irresponsibility? Instead of eschewing children due to the belief that therapy without parental involvement is futile, what if we embrace them with open minds, hands, and hearts?* Original programmers may be best, but secondary programming is absolutely useful. How many times have we heard parents either proudly or with chagrin say, "Well, I don't know where they learned that, certainly not from me!" Our brains, especially the mind of a child, are malleable, adaptive, and not static (Steinberg, 2017). It seems the field has focused so much on the idea that parents need to be the ones to do the work first that we have forgotten those who are not in a place to work this way. The following scenarios are some that have crossed my path or paths of my colleagues who work with children.

I have a dear friend who works with kids in the foster care system. He rarely can work with his parents. I have another friend who owns a foster care agency and is currently receiving a grant to work with unaccompanied minors, refugee children separated from their parents. Right now, there are thousands of these children in the state I live in, along with other bordering states with completely severed families. I am hoping to work with them in some capacity. There are also parents who, for whatever reasons, refuse, despite being asked and advised that it would be best for their children if they participate in therapy, will not do so. I have colleagues who have experienced clients calling an Uber for their children to attend sessions. Often, divorced parents work to make sure the alternate parent can have nothing to do with their child's therapy and so forgo their own involvement. They say it is imperative that the other "parent not interfere" with their child's treatment. I have time and again witnessed white-collar professional parents relay that their busy schedules restrict them from attending therapy with their child. These are just a few reasons that parents might be unable or unwilling to work collaboratively with their children.

On the other hand, it is often possible to get the parent's buy-in for involvement, and whenever we can, it is wise to continue to do so. When we cannot, it is imperative to do whatever we can to provide the best care possible. This book endeavors to provide the clinician with the knowledge and skill to do so.

As I have heard the troubling comments from clinicians above, I have thought through where these may be coming from and would like to take a look at some plausible subtext:

> I was very uncomfortable working with kids as a new therapist and did not have much training or direction in this type of work. It was relieving when I was able to choose a different population.
>
> From my learning as a family therapist, parents have to be involved or lasting change is impossible and at the very least improbable. We are better spending time on other efforts.

It is time for us to question our mantras. This is the way of our predecessors in the field. It is helpful to remember the field of Marriage and Family Therapy is relatively young, and there is still much to explore. The newness of our practice often strikes me when I hear Terry D. Hargrave reminiscing of his time spent face-to-face with Carl Whitaker, Jay Hayley, and Chloe Madanes. I appreciate what Salvador Minuchin said of Jay Hayley.

"Jay was forever pushing the envelope, testing the limits of new ideas— explorations that bore his imprint of being clear, over-inclusive, and challenging. . . . He was always available to his students. Even at the end of the day, he could be seen surrounded by young people, as a peripatetic Greek philosopher without a toga" (Baker, 2010).

As previously stated, every great teacher (or learner) has the qualities of curiosity, skepticism, and humility. As we look at our various opportunities to approach work with children, fortunately, the top-down approach is not the only way to create change in the family system. Marriage and Family therapy touts that when any member of the family system gets healthy, it is impactful (Balswick, 2008). This is true of kids as well.

Let's pause for a moment to think about the impact children can have on our own families. For those of us with children, grandchildren, nieces, or nephews, can we think about a time when the kids in our system have taught us something valuable? Would we be so bold to say that our children have never brought us insight from their healthy views of the world? I can recall plenty of times when my kids ushered me toward a healthier way of relating. "Mom, why do you sound so mad at me and then sound really happy when you answer the phone?" "Mom, don't be scared; God will take care of us."

The cybernetic nature of family therapy highlights how family members get caught in "dysfunctional feedback loops-acting and reacting to each other in unhelpful ways" (Nichols, 2009). Restoration Therapy acknowledges this in a fresh and remarkably applicable way and then gets to work detecting and highlighting these exact patterns. After this occurs, the therapist and patient alike can recognize unhealthy patterns visually, cognitively, and emotionally. After the client learns how to reverse the dysfunctional feedback loops into functional feedback loops, they are on their way from pain to peace.

My mother tells a story about when my daughter, still a toddler, greatly impacted her. My mother was struggling with depression and low self-worth. My daughter was two years old and excited to spend some time at grandma's house; while she climbed the steps leading to my Mom's front porch, she began shouting self-affirmations and that which was the truth. Step one, "I beautiful," step two, "I wonderful," step three, "I strong," step four, "I will grow big!" step five, "I will be a lovely lady!!" When she reached the top step, my Mom picked her up and kissed both of her chubby little cheeks. This action reinforced my daughter's belief that her self-talk was all the truest of realities, and it did not only reinforce this reality for my daughter, but it strengthened it for her grandmother as well. My daughter led her grandma toward health in this instance. It did not harm my daughter to lead here in the slightest; instead, it solidified her own positive identity.

This story still brings tears to my Mom's eyes when she tells it. She was reminded in a dark time of doubt of the truth of her intrinsic worth and value. She was able to take joy in these truths in a personally meaningful way while my daughter shouted them out in gleeful assurance. We are all born with power. At two and a half years old, my daughter, Michele, spoke functional into dysfunctional and spurred on the wheels of positive change within our family system. Kids are often underestimated in the therapeutic room. They are marginalized when they have a unique ability to bring profound truths and healing to a family.

Approaching critical scientific thinking requires curiosity, skepticism, and humility (Myers & DeWall, 2010). In this helping field, we rightfully are *curious* about how best to help children learn to deal with their pain effectively. We are *skeptical* that lasting change can only be found for kids whose parents are willing to take the lead. We are also *skeptical* that kids don't have the power to effect change in the system. Yet, we maintain our traditional belief as marriage and family therapists that relational dynamics are a sort of eco-system, where each part impacts the others. We are *humble* in that we readily concede we do not know it all. We see this field in part but not in its entirety. There is still much to be explored. We are questioners by the nature of our profession, remaining open to new ideas to more effectively help those in need. We are also *humble* enough to get down on the floor and often on our knees to minister to a small child's needs. In our humility, we seek to empower them.

We acknowledge that all have a certain amount of power, and whenever we use it to empower others, we are giving some of our own away. This was evidenced in the biblical story of the woman touching Jesus's garment in (Luke 8:46, NIV). He said, "someone touched me; I know that power has gone out from me." This never feels entirely comfortable at the moment. As part of the helping profession, we also have a particular faith that comes from experience. Time and again, we see that what we give seems to return to us, and often in greater measure. The task of helping little ones is a worthwhile effort.

One of my curious, skeptical, and humble mentors made a great point in this regard. Often, as is the case in session, we listen and observe and our patients both show and tell us what they need to heal. My doctorate involved a mentorship with H. Norman Wright. He is a longtime professor, therapist, and author of over 90 books. He asked me to guess where he received the best education. He attended some great schools, including Westmont, Pepperdine, and Fuller. I assumed Fuller Seminary with a smile as I knew we shared this common training ground. He winked and agreed he had indeed attended some great schools, but his answer was not what I expected. He stated the answer directly and confidently. "My clients. They are and have always been my most excellent teachers."

The Client Our Greatest Teacher—A Little Child Will Lead Them

Kids can teach us valuable lessons. I have time and again witnessed children incite significant change in their family system. Several case studies follow, which supports this "upside-down approach" to what we were taught. The teaching that parents are supposed to lead the system, not children. It is interesting to note that the ancient biblical text of (Isaiah 11:6, NIV) states, "The wolf will live with the lamb, the leopard will lie down with the goat, the calf and the lion and the yearling together and a little child will lead them." This verse is, of course, prophetically speaking about the Messiah who will bring peace to a world full of conflict. Currently, instead of calm, there is a clamor in our relationships. Fighting family members could be likened to wolves, leopards, and lions devouring lambs, goats, and calves.

Instead of living harmoniously, we live with the temptation to let our fight or flight instincts reign as we fear our sense of identity or safety. It is poignant the animals mentioned above in these verses; all have intense fight or flight responses. This writing speaks of a confident hope that these "fighters" and "fleers" might live in harmony one day, laying aside the victimizer victim roles. Interestingly in this effort of restoration, "a little child will lead them."

There is profound wisdom in the symbolism and message of this metaphor. There is something beautifully innocent and honest about children. Children are yet vulnerable, uncovered by the hardened shell of various harmful coping mechanisms. They are often more willing to try new things, and they learn quickly. They tend to be brave and are continually forging new paths, both neurologically and relationally. Their examples are compelling. This book includes fictionalized narratives but somewhat similar (less any identifying information) to children whose stories are tattooed on my mind and heart. Children whose hard work I fiercely admire. I hope we can begin to honor children in more significant ways in the field of family therapy. We must push past our preconceived ideas to create room for them in this wonderful healing field where we reside. This book will prove useful for people in the psychotherapeutic helping professions who work with both individual children and their families. Additionally, secondary target audiences are parents and elementary school educators.

References

Baker, M. (2010). *The power of two – Revisiting Jay Haley through the voice of Madeleine Richeport-Haley*, Vol. 30, No. 3. The M.H. Erickson Foundation Newsletter, https://moam.info/jay-haley-and-madeleine-richeport-haley_5a321e631723dd569788cf64.html

Balswick, J. O. (2008). *The family: A Christian perspective on the contemporary home.* Baker Academic.

Kaslow, F. W. (1996). *Handbook of relational diagnosis and dysfunctional family patterns.* Wiley.

Minuchin, S., & Fishman, H. C. (1998). *Family therapy techniques.* Harvard University Press.

Myers, David G., & DeWall, C. N. (2010). *Exploring psychology.* Worth Publishers.

Napier, A. Y., & Whitaker, C. (1978). *The family crucible: The intense experience of family therapy.* Harper Perennial.

Nichols, M. P. (2009). *Inside family therapy: A case study in family healing.* Allyn & Bacon.

Steinberg, L. D. (2017). *Adolescence.* McGraw-Hill Education.

1 Helping Kids Find Relief and Healing

An Overview of the Restoration Therapy Model

Her Mom carefully pried her daughter's small fingers one by one off of the car door handle. She continued to cling as tightly as she possibly could; the skin under her nailbeds had gone from pink to ghostly white. A great wave of fear enveloped her, threatening to knock her over, face first, into the pebbled black asphalt. Her stomach churned, and her little knees trembled. She was being torn away from the safety of the family car and shuddered at the realization she would be separated from her Mom within mere minutes. Through a blur of hot tears, she looked at the large and looming burnt-orange brick school building ahead of her. She hated first grade! At that thought, her feet seemed to take on a life of their own and began to run. After the first few steps, they were halted by a firm yank on her crisp white sweater-wrapped arm. Defeated, she settled into her Mom's grip. She knew she was going to be scolded. She didn't want to be disobedient, but the emotions felt so overwhelming at times that she wondered if she really had a choice.

A similar story played out many a morning for this golden-haired, brown-eyed little girl. She was well-loved by her parents and teachers. Feeling loved wasn't the issue. She listened to her Mom and Dad whispering at night, trying to find strategies to alleviate her fear; she knew her teachers discussed her in their meetings. Her Mom began to volunteer in the classroom, but on the days and hours she couldn't be there, there was no improvement; in fact, they all wondered if it made matters worse. The teacher gave her awards at lunchtime if she hadn't cried yet and made a big deal out of it in front of the class. Attention was not what she wanted. She wasn't seeking a spotlight; it only made her more uncomfortable. She just wanted to disappear, to go home and be with her Mom. At the time, it was an unsolved mystery for everyone involved.

As I write this narrative, it is astounding to me how all of the emotions pour back into my being as if I am transported back to that moment. The little girl in the white sweater was me. She still lives in me, although much has changed. The mystery has been solved, she is now understood, validated; she can see the truth and therefore respond differently. I now know the steps to move from pain to peace. For this, I am grateful; My only regret

DOI: 10.4324/9781003025504-1

is that it took so long. I often tell clients that shame and regret are different animals. Shame has a quality of stagnation, wallowing if you will. Regret inspires forward movement. Regret is a change agent. My hope is for this book to help bring immediate relief to kids in pain. There is no good reason to eschew children and make them wait until they are older. The four objectives of Restoration Therapy are remarkably effective and adaptable to working with children. The straightforward, understandable approach has been bringing relief to both clients and clinicians for years. The therapy model is pragmatic and provides a roadmap that therapists can learn and follow. For a more in-depth look at the model, practice, and overview of Restoration Therapy, I recommend the book *Restoration Therapy: Understanding and Guiding Healing in Marriage and Family Therapy* by Terry D. Hargrave and Franz Pfitzer.

Brief Description of the Restoration Therapy Model

The theoretical approach of RT is rooted in family systems. The systemic nature accounts for relational dynamics at play. It carefully considers relational and family context when working with a client. The therapist diligently searches to understand what part of the patient's pain is stemming from discordant relationships or how the greater community surrounding the client might be impactful in helpful or harmful ways. RT also analyzes the impact of early bonding and the family of origin. It carefully considers occurrences of a breach of love or trustworthiness. Love and trustworthiness are the two pillars of healthy attachment (Hargrave, 2019). Jonathon Bowlby's theory of attachment explored the bonds between primary care givers and children. He noted the importance of healthy attachment and the detrimental outcomes caused by poor attachment (Bowlby, 1988). If a child feels pervasively unsafe or unloved, it is indicative of an attachment injury that needs repairing. Thus, in addition to taking a family systems approach, RT is also rooted in Attachment Theory.

Furthermore, RT believes that love and trust can best be learned best in a "here and now" (Hargrave & Pfitzer, 2011). experience. Therefore, the theory and practice of RT are experiential in nature. The therapist not only works to listen and understand the origin of the pain and resulting behavior, but they also challenge inaccurate beliefs the clients are holding and implement new patterns of change in the therapy session. The therapist looks to observe maladaptive processes which are occurring in session and seeks to disrupt the patterns in vivo. Lastly, RT has been called "the new contextual theory." It adheres to the idea that there needs to be a sense of fairness and balance within relationships for health to occur both interpersonally and intrapersonally (Hargrave & Pfitzer, 2011). There is much attention paid to intrapersonal and interpersonal patterns that have developed. RT touts that life begins and is lived out in patterns (Hargrave, 2019). As humans develop cognitively and emotionally, patterns form. These patterns can become problematic. The RT therapist is adept at identifying these unhealthy patterns and helping the client create new ones through a four-step process, including mindfulness. RT extrapolates from the best of various theories: family systems, attachment, experiential, and contextual. RT then masterfully organizes and synthesizes them into an unmatched pragmatic theory of its own.

Overview of the Four Objectives of Restoration

The four objectives for an RT therapist can be easily understood and stated. They are as follows: 1.) Identifying and understanding the pain cycle, 2.) Determining the emotionally regulating truth, 3.) Identifying and understanding the Peace Cycle, 4.) Practicing the Four Steps (Hargrave, 2019).

In moving from educator to therapist, I had a unique experience. I was used to planning for a class. Each day, I would lay out goals and objectives, and planned the lesson in that way. When I tried to prepare for a session with a client, I found it to be much more ambiguous than lesson planning. Before my introduction to RT, I was confused about how to create treatment goals and objectives. Now with RT, I am able to develop goals and objectives. This allows me to track and measure forward or backward movement. Effective therapists should be able to assess if a client is progressing or digressing quickly. In working with student interns outside of RT, treatment planning appears unclear to them. In the educational world, teachers are often required to write the students' daily objectives on the whiteboard. When classes end, they can simply look at the whiteboard and know if they have done their job by meeting the objective. For therapists, especially traditional play therapists, measuring treatment objectives has been a nebulous effort. RT provides a relieving roadmap for both the therapist and client. Clients can easily detect when therapists are all over the map and find it disconcerting.

This particular book is aimed at helping children through using the RT process. It is unique in its application but adheres closely to the four objectives of RT. The following paragraphs will uncover each step in greater detail and provide examples of how to move through the process, specifically with children. The last section of the book provides step by step practical application. Instead of educational lesson plans, the term "session plans" has been coined and created. These will help clinicians get a jump start on adapting RT to therapeutic work with children.

Objective One: Identifying and Understanding the Pain Cycle

Identifying and understanding the pain cycle can be applied to children in various ways. The first order of business is to get a glimpse into the story of the child's damaged identity and or safety. The therapist asks not "what is wrong with you?" but rather, "what has happened to you?" Even more specifically, the clinician seeks to see and understand when and by whom have they experienced feeling either unloved or unsafe? The clinician explores the child's past and current attachment relationships for an attachment injury. After discovering the answers to these questions, the therapist can better understand the child's coping behaviors. The coping behaviors are more overt than attachment injuries or the painful feelings children often silently carry. Typically, coping behaviors are, at least in part, the presenting problems that brought the child into the therapy room. As a case in point, the story from my childhood displayed my coping behaviors vividly. I coped through escape and control (attempting to run away or control my environment by keeping my Mom by my side.) These coping strategies were noticeable, but the more profound breach in safety was not easily identified, hence the unsolved mystery. An effective therapist needs to look underneath the presenting problem to help second-order change occur.

Interestingly, when observing a child coping through escaping and controlling behaviors, the therapist can be relatively sure the child is suffering from a safety violation. On the other hand, when the child is coping through blaming or shaming behaviors, it is equally indicative of an identity violation (an actual or perceived lack of love.) Once the child's painful emotions can be discovered, the clinician can match each feeling with a coinciding coping behavior. These are patterns that develop early on. The circular design is what RT defines as the pain cycle. The pain cycle can be delineated with a cognitive map, which can transform into an innovative visual construct to help the child clearly see, identify, and learn their patterned ways of dealing with conflict.

To summarize, the first objective of Restoration Therapy is defining and understanding the pain. To get to the destination, it is essential to start with the more observable coping strategies the client displays. This is where the therapist observes the coping behaviors and, like a police dog, follows the scent to uncover the actual perpetrator. The coping or acting out that the clients present with is symptomatic and will inevitably lead to their pain. Discovering the source of their pain is the first goal (Hargrave, 2019). The following example illustrates why this is the crucial first objective.

A dear professor from my undergraduate university is currently going through what is nearing six months of testing to discover an internal bleed source. They know he is bleeding because he is pale, weak; he has low blood pressure and other indicative symptoms. He seems to have had every kind of scan imaginable; he was made to swallow a pill-sized camera and has been in and out of hospitals. Sadly, as of yet, they have been unsuccessful in finding the source. Therefore, he is forced to undergo weekly transfusions and is frequently hospitalized due to pain and malaise. The doctors are chasing his symptoms, looking for the epicenter of his pain to detect the bleed source.

Similarly, as Restoration Therapists, this is the first order of business. For the child, acting out and coping are symptomatic of a deeper source of pain. If the source is not discovered, the therapist remains stuck in a frustrating loop of treating the symptoms without finding the problem. As with my professor, as soon as they identify the source, the problem can be remedied.

Objective Two: Identifying the Truth

During the second objective, the therapist's work is to help the child identify and understand truths (primary emotions that are positive in nature.) These truths are most often in direct contrast to the painful and patterned emotions experienced from an actual or perceived lack of love or safety. For example, if a child has experienced significant and perpetual breaches in trustworthiness when conflict occurs, he/she may feel powerless. The antithesis to the pain of powerlessness is powerful or empowered. Because it is a true statement that each person, child, or adult is endowed with a certain measure of power, the therapist can guide the child into realizing their intrinsic power. When the child can affirm and recognize their power's reality, their emotional state changes, it is regulated, and they can be freed from reactivity. In the author's narrative, her "feet took on a life of their own and started running." The reactivity was the flight response. Had someone let her know the truth, that she had power, she could use her voice, ask good questions, and clarify when she felt confused; it would have initiated a sense of calm.

Her parents and teachers indeed were on her side. What might have happened if, instead of running away and becoming catastrophically anxious, she stayed engaged in the conversation and moment by speaking up and letting her concerns be known? The work of this second step involves intentional guidance on the part of the therapist to aid the child in moving away from false narratives, which ignite reactivity. In this teachable space of calm, the child can understand and assimilate the need to pause and take care of their painful feelings (Siegal & Bryson, 2012). This involves mindfully moving away from negative self-talk into the truths of their safety and identity and basking in this new reality.

Objective Three: The Peace Cycle

A most profound intervention that RT provides the therapist with is what is called the Peace Cycle. As with the Pain Cycle, the therapist can help the child by using flashcards or drawings to create a visual representation of their patterned painful feelings and consequent coping methods. In exploring and defining the Peace Cycle, the therapist guides, in the same way, to help the child construct a visual, cognitive map of the child's truths and the subsequent actions which follow when the child is living out of the truth. For instance, when the child, who typically feels powerless, considers their power, rather than needing to escape or disengage, they are empowered to engage in a productive conversation. It is the understanding of RT that children are typically good at heart but misbehave when they are in the reactive pain cycle (Hargrave, 2019). If the clinician can help them recognize and honor their intrinsic value, and that much about life can be trusted, including themselves, reactivity falls away. This allows their good-heartedness to shine through.

Objective Four: Practice the Four Steps

After walking through the first three objectives, the child has gained insight into their rooted pain and reactivity patterns. They are armed with newly realized truths about their value and sense of safety and agency. Consequentially they are ready to put it all together into four easily understood and easy to practice steps that will lead them out of pain and into peace.

The four steps of moving from pain to peace are as follows:

Step One: Say what you feel.
Step Two: Say what you normally do.
Step Three: Say the truth.
Step Four: Say what you will do differently.

First, the therapist moves toward helping the client practice validating their pain. They can do this by simply saying it out loud. "I feel like I don't matter." Next, they work to slow down the typical lightning-quick leap to reactivity. The child can do this by telling themselves what they typically do when they feel the painful emotion. "When I feel like I don't matter, I normally get hyper and start talking too much." As the child moves into Step Three, they engage the reasoning part of their brain to remind themselves of the truth and, in so doing, tend to their heart; the heart calms, and emotions settle. Step Three may sound something like, "The truth is that I do matter. I matter a lot to my Mom, my sister; I matter to God and myself." A resulting sense of peace leads to Step Four.

In Step Four, they say what they will do differently. "Instead of getting hyper and talking too much, I will sit quietly and be a good listener." Step Four is naturally born from the sense of stability that Step Three brings. Consequentially, positive actions rather than negative reactivity will naturally occur. This concise linear path helps the child know precisely how to move forward effectively. It is a fantastic process to observe a child move from pain to peace. Chapter 5 will further detail creative ways to help kids remember the four steps, including a song. It is imperative to spend time working through these steps with the client. Insight is excellent but too often provides fleeting relief. Lasting brain-change only occurs after the child is well-practiced.

Imagine coaching tennis and simply describing the correct form and movement to a child and then sending them to a tournament while expecting them actually to win a match. This is arguably a ridiculous expectation. The beauty of working with children is that they are willing to practice, practice, practice! Especially if they are met with creative, fun methods of recalling and implementing the four steps. Putting the four steps within a playful context including, arts, crafts, body movements, and music, is sure to sear it in their memories and practice. The Fourth Objective of RT, The Four Steps, is the crown on top of the RT process. These steps provide practical guidance and a clear path forward for the child and therapists. The RT approach was created to help patients, but it may be true that the even greater passion for RT founders is to help provide equipped and excellent therapists. The following narrative illustrates the void that RT seeks to fill for new or unsure clinicians about engaging in therapy with children.

A Directive Approach: Bringing Direction and Relief to Clinicians

Throughout the past few years, I have had the occasion to speak to therapist colleagues about feeling directionless in their work with children. As people have become aware of this book which offers a structured approach to work with children, it has provided more conversations. Although some enjoy standard play therapy practice, many find it problematic. Just this week, a new therapist with a desire to help children relayed her experience at a recent play therapy training.

> I was in shock as I looked around at 300 people. The facilitating thera-
> pist showed a video of two six-year-olds arguing over a toy and "letting"
> the children "figure it out" Every part of my brain was screaming "just
> show them how!" One child was a bully. The other sat silently while
> the therapy room was destroyed by the first child sweeping all the toys
> off the shelves. The therapist just sat and watched. As I observed other
> attendees nod their heads in agreement and take notes, I felt as if we
> were buying into a notion like the Emperor's New Clothes.

I recall frantically searching through my supervisor's bins of toys to find some that a six-year-old boy would likely enjoy. I was a brand-new thera-pist preparing to see my first client, who was a child. I had always wanted to work with children. I imagined gaining rapport with him would not be difficult. However, I was still anxious and unsure of what this new sort of experience with a pediatric patient might look like. How was I to help a vulnerable child in a painful place? I desired practical direction, ideas, and skills.

Inadvertently harming a child or causing one ounce of unnecessary addi-tional pain to his/her life was unthinkable. I was already seeing adults and just getting used to them. I was still hyper-vigilant about everything that I was doing and saying. Adults are bigger, stronger, I thought. If I made a mistake with something, I did or said they could reason and fight back or against me. An adult could fire me at will. This thought brought me peculiar relief.

I had worked tirelessly to enter the field as a helper and still felt sorely inexperienced. My confidence was small, and I was highly self-critical. I was overly conscious of every word or facial expression I naturally wanted to release in session.

I cautiously hid my natural response and quickly locked up any rogue twitch or curve of my mouth. I was aware of all of this while trying to hear my clients' every word or observe any slight change in their body language. On the outside, I calmly nodded my head, trying to mirror my client. One of my biggest complaints to a close colleague was that I couldn't feel my face after consecutive sessions. We still laugh about it. It was a clear somatic response from my internal battle of hiding any possible forbidden facial expression. I was trying too hard. I needed to relax and allow myself to meet my clients with authentic responses while being therapeutically appropriate. I was exhausted each night after a day of seeing people.

I was also learning self-care and letting go of client issues instead of carrying them home with me. I was a bundle of nerves, unsure of nearly every approach to the varied nuances of therapy. Imagine if I was this apprehensive about working with adults; what the prospect of working with my first pediatric client felt like?

Thankfully my supervisor, Dr. Bailey, was and is a remarkable person. She is knowledgeable, available, supportive, and humble. I am eternally grateful for her example. Being a beginning therapist is a painfully vulnerable experience. It is difficult and necessary to ask for help when first entering the field. It is embarrassing and painful to make mistakes. As a supervisor, Dr. Bailey modeled what RT considers to be the two pillars of a healthy relationship. She was *trustworthy* and *valued me (loving)*. In return, I trusted her and felt safe to be vulnerable in moments when I thought I had failed or needed instruction.

I am a relatively independent person who doesn't typically need much attention. However, as a new therapist, I needed to ask questions; I needed to know what was reasonable, appropriate, professional when to quell or release my expression. Despite my supervisor's gracious reassurance, I struggled with feeling like a bother. I recall desiring written instruction on how to work with particular populations and how to meet treatment goals. I longed for something similar to what I had as a teacher, not exactly lesson plans but session plans! If I had more precise direction, I wouldn't have to worry about demanding too much of my supervisor's time, and I could feel confident.

I currently have the honor of supervising interns, and I think most in the field remember their own experiences of being new. There is a hearty agreement that an easy-to-follow therapeutic framework, along with a supportive supervisor, is invaluable. It is anxiety-producing to feel lost or directionless. This nerve-wracking feeling of being lost, particularly in the predominately non-directive play therapy world, gave rise to applying the RT model to work with kids.

Interns and supervisees tend to be inundated with, to quote Mary Ainsworth out of context, "strange situations." Perhaps it is part of earning their stripes, or God in his wisdom, allowing them to experience unorthodox scenarios when they have someone to run to for help. Whatever the reason is, the truth is that it is excruciating for a new therapist to lack clear direction. Restoration Play Therapy will provide hope to therapists who feel unsure, moving them into the peaceful assurance that they can be armed with a roadmap of how to help most effectively. The latter part of the book provides practical step-by-step help through "session plans." They are innovative, therapeutically researched, sound, and enjoyable.

Structured With Room to Create

After soaking up science, history, and therapy theory, the day comes when it is time to apply what the books teach. Many excellent methods seem to be lacking a bridge or playbook for practical application. My desire is for this book to be practically applicable to help new therapists in their healing work.

As a previous English teacher, I taught young writers how to create and format poetry. I found my creative students would bristle at the idea of having to adhere to specific forms or structures like sonnets, limericks, or haikus. They "just wanted to write," they said. My more linear students bemoaned having to "make stuff up," they visited my desk repeatedly, wanting more detailed instructions. They counted their syllables tediously, and the few things about poetry that gave them pleasure or relief were the idea that they could understand what a quatrain or cinquain was because they were sure that they could count numbers of lines in a bunch. They could also practically understand the meanings of alliteration and assonance. These objective rules gave them a foundation to build on.

It could be argued that all things beautiful and practical have both structure and art. Restoration Therapy has both, and for whatever type of learner we are as a therapist or a client, Restoration Therapy makes good sense and is enjoyable to practice. The four objectives are like four solidly built walls of a dance studio. The clinicians and clients can dance within the walls using their style, movement, and music choice, yet feel secure, assured that they would not fall off a suspended swaying platform. Restoration Therapy is neither nebulous nor stifling but rather has clearly stated objectives with plenty of room for creativity, making both sides of our brain happier.

A Summary of the Theory and Four Goals of Restoration Therapy

The general roadmap of Restoration Therapy can be described as follows:

Parents almost always seek therapeutic intervention for their children due to conflict of some kind. With conflict comes emotional pain caused by feelings of being unsafe or unloved. Conflict and pain are bedfellows. To deal with the pain brought on by conflict, kids, like adults, turn to various destructive coping mechanisms. These coping mechanisms fall under the four distinct umbrellas of blame, shame, control, and escape. While working with the child, the therapist begins to move through the four established goals of Restoration Therapy: 1.) Define and understand the pain, 2.) Identify the truth, 3.) Emotionally regulate using child's truths and 4.) Mindful Practice.

In moving through these established goals, the child can gain insight and be able to achieve successful change through practicing the truth. In knowing these core truths about themselves, they can be set free from emotional and relational bondage.

This roadmap is akin to a treasure map! Armed with a pragmatic path forward, the therapist can help kids find a sense of personal and relational peace. It is not possible to lead others well unless there is an understanding of the path forward and through a client's pain. There needs to be an awareness of where the pitfalls and traps typically lie. If kids have fallen into a pit or are caught in a trap, the clinician needs to be able to identify the sort of trap they are in and know well the way to lead them out.

Restoration Therapy: Playing Their Way From Pain to Peace, trains therapists to determine the kinds of painful pits in which kids are desperately trapped. They then can see how children are ineffectively attempting to break free but only sinking deeper. This education is imperative. People who are uneducated regarding how to break free from quicksand often perish if they fall into it. However, those who are educated can easily survive a fall into a quagmire; it isn't an easy effort to break free from quicksand; it requires first learning and then practicing counter-intuitive action. An informed person understands that they will stay afloat by holding still instead of obeying their natural response.

Although "holding still" may not be adequate to break free from emotional pain, counter-intuitive action is needed. Just like any person, young or old, can be educated about how to survive quicksand, so can both children and adults be equipped, and empowered to survive emotional pain, and therefore, thrive in relationships rather than perishing.

Helping children move from pain to peace is a worthy effort and one that can be carried out with clarity and skill. The following chapters explain in greater detail the path to helping children find relief from the symptoms and origin of their pain. This work's structure is somewhat unique in that it uses case studies, vignettes, and personal stories to explain the theory and approach. There are eighteen session plans at the end of the book to clearly guide the therapist in implementing RT with children.

References

Bowlby, J. (1988). *A secure base*. Basic Books.

Hargrave, T. D. (2019). *Advances and techniques in restoration therapy*. Routledge and Taylor & Francis Group.

Hargrave, T. D., & Pfitzer, F. (2011). *Restoration therapy: Understanding and guiding healing in marriage and family therapy*. Routledge.

Siegal, D. J., & Bryson, T. P. (2012). *The whole-brain child: 12 Revolutionary strategies to nurture your child's developing mind. Bantam books trade PBK*. New York: Bantam Books.

2 Fight or Flight? Let's Fight!

My Mom once told me a story about the fight or flight response that she recalled hearing from a pastor. It got me thinking about my work with children and their ability to soldier through conflict and often transcend the fight or flight response through mindfulness. It went something like this:

The Lying Lizard

"I decided to take my three children to an Olympic-sized swimming pool to practice holding their breath and simply to become better all-around swimmers. The kids jumped into the pool when we got there, giggling and splashing. When it was time to focus more on form and fortitude in the water, I had the idea to make it a little competitive."

"Okay, kids, I hollered so they could hear me. Here is the deal! Whoever can swim from one side of the pool to the other without taking a breath gets the biggest ice-cream cone on the way home." My two boys were 10 and 8, and my daughter was six years old at the time. Jumping up out down, with excitement at the challenge, they jockeyed for position. It was decided they would start in age order, oldest to youngest. My 10-year-old took a deep exaggerated breath and plunged in. He started strong, but halfway through, the pool's length surfaced for air and stopped. He splashed the water in frustration, swam to the side, and climbed out, glaring at the ground.

Before I could say a word to him, my second son splashed in and was on his way. He looked confident and pressed past the middle, but a quarter of the way before the end, he popped, up gulping in the air, and immediately began talking trash to his older brother that at least he had made it further than him. He climbed out, puffing his chest, and strutted past his brother like the little turkey he was acting.

My daughter ran up to me and beckoned me to bend down to her level so she could speak quietly in my ear. "Dad! I really want to win." "I smiled and said "okay then!" Let me tell you a secret, and this secret is going to make you win if you can trust me. Do you trust me to tell you the truth?" She looked at me intently eye-to-eye and nodded her head firmly in the affirmative and with an air of finality. "Okay," I whispered. There is a little lizard that lives

DOI: 10.4324/9781003025504-2

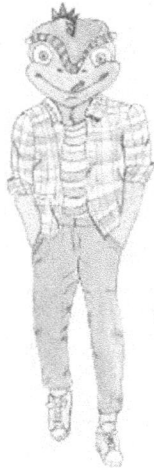

Figure 2.1 Lenny the Lying Lizard

in all of our brains, and this lizard is a liar. You are going to take a breath, plenty big enough to get you across that pool, but this lizard is going to tell you that you are going to die if you don't take a breath before you get to the other side. I want you to remember he is a liar, and don't you listen to him. Just keep swimming. Remember I've watched you practice and I know you can do this. She nodded again with steely strength in her eyes. She walked to the pool and jumped in.

She started strong; she passed the middle, still strong, she finished the final quarter, slowed for a minute as if she was thinking but continued. She sprang up at the end, gulped in some air, and with a big grin hollered up at me, "Dad! That lizard is LOUD!!" We all cheered, and later she welcomed the biggest ice-cream cone with a memorable grin of satisfaction at a job very well done.

Current brain research establishes that the fight or flight response follows real or perceived threats. Whether in physical or emotional pain, the brain signals this response, and to self-protect, we launch into understandable yet destructive ways of coping (Hanna, 2014). There are four types of unhelpful coping methods that we tend to fall into blame, shame, control, and escape. There are varied ways of acting these out. Attachment theory suggests that to thrive, there needs to be a secure attachment bond (Bowlby, 1988). When feelings of being unloved or unsafe arise, our fundamental need for secure attachment is threatened. Typically, when there is a threat of being unloved, children respond by blaming others or shaming themselves. When there is a threat signaling that things are unsafe, the typical coping response is control or escape.

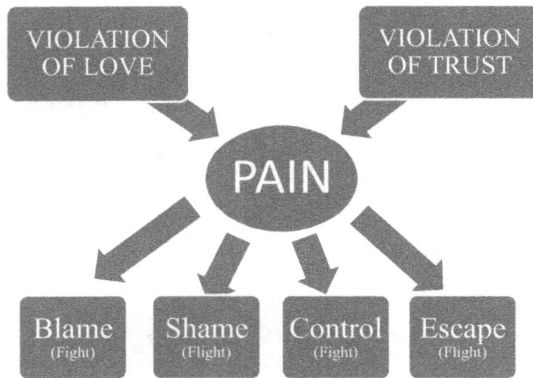

Figure 2.2 Origin of Pain and Coping Responses

The fight response during a love violation is blame, and during a safety violation it is control (Hargrave, 2019). Blame and control are an attempt to take action to quell these intolerable core emotions of feeling unloved or unsafe. This chapter delves into how blame and control are often exhibited when children attempt to fight off emotional turmoil. A clear understanding of these responses aids the therapist in identifying the underlying pain. The chapter provides case studies and vignettes to help answer practical questions of implementation.

It is interesting to note that in the biblical story of Genesis 3, we can observe from our earliest recorded writings that human nature has ever sought to alleviate the pain of relational conflict by reacting through blame, shame, control, and escape. Adam and Eve were told to enjoy everything in the Garden of Eden, except for the tree of the knowledge of good and evil. When the cold-blooded serpent stirred up and created conflict, they chose to handle it through "control," taking things into their own hands. The narrative shows us how they responded with shame, control, escape, and blame.

> "You will not certainly die," the serpent said to the woman. "For God knows that when you eat from it, your eyes will be opened, and you will be like God, knowing good and evil." When the woman saw that the fruit of the tree was good for food and pleasing to the eye and also desirable for gaining wisdom, she took some and ate it. She also gave some to her husband, who was with her, and he ate it. Then the eyes of both of them were opened, and they realized they were naked; so, they sewed fig leaves together and made coverings for themselves. Then the man and his wife heard the sound of the Lord God as he was walking in the garden in the cool of the day, and they hid from the Lord God

among the trees of the garden. But the Lord God called to the man, "Where are you?" He answered, "I heard you in the garden, and I was afraid because I was naked; so, I hid." And he said, "Who told you that you were naked? Have you eaten from the tree that I commanded you not to eat from?" The man said, "The woman you put here with me— she gave me some fruit from the tree, and I ate it." Then the Lord God said to the woman, "What is this you have done?" The woman said, "The serpent deceived me, and I ate."

(Genesis 3:4–13, NIV)

We see in the text that Eve decided to take *control* by eating the apple, and then Adam did likewise. They, in turn, "realized they were naked and became *ashamed*." The text illustrates how they attempted to cope through *control* again when they came up with a plan to fix the problem by sewing fig leaves together to cover themselves. When they saw this wasn't working according to their plan, they *escaped* by hiding from God. When God began to question them, Adam immediately *blamed* both God and Eve by saying, "The woman you put here with me gave me some fruit." Eve, in turn, *blamed* the serpent saying, "The serpent deceived me." This concept of conflict creating pain in our brain and subsequently causing us to move into the fight or flight response is ancient and intrinsic to human nature.

What is often called the Lizard or Reptilian Brain is what Paul MacLean explained as the area of the human brain which control behaviors preserving survival (1990). It drives primal desires, and is part of the limbic system which contains the amygdala. The Lizard part of our brain is essential and instinctive, quickly springing into action in order to protect us needed. like a lizard; as long as we catch it, it can be handled swiftly and easily kicked out of the house. In short, we can take charge of a lizard. In the hierarchical power structure, the mindful brain is the "boss" of the lizard! In Arizona, where I live, we get used to seeing a lot of lizards scurrying around our desert landscape and often our homes! This is precisely why my husband gets a big kick out of me screaming and running from a gecko who may have decided to join me in the shower or, heaven forbid, mistakes my leg for a tree branch. Sometimes lizards can cause quite the start, but the reality is that they are benign creatures who, when bid to flee, don't have much of a choice but to do so.

Restoration Therapy helps us to identify our core emotions and then challenge our unhelpful responses that so often stem from that which is not true. Imagine if the ability to recognize the "Lizard" for what it was would change our actions. As we read, play with, and observe our patients, the first goal is to find the painful emotion. We often do this by following the coping behaviors and categorizing them into blame, shame, control, or escape. In the following case vignette, this child has the fight response when in pain. Let's take note to see if this child tends to move toward blame or control. Once we identify this, we can explore the painful feelings behind it.

Restoration Play Therapy has created four interactive coping characters to illustrate these fight and flight responses children use when they are dysregulated. They are helpful tools and come in the form of puppets, toys, drawings. There are also songs and stories written about them.

The Coping Characters

The four characters are Brutus the Blaming Badger, Contessa the Controlling Cow, Sharla the Shameful Sheep, and Eddie the Escape Goat. I use the characters pictured below and or puppets of the following animals in session to act out various personally applicable scenarios to the pediatric patient.

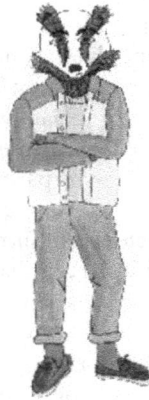

Figure 2.3 Brutus the Blaming Badger

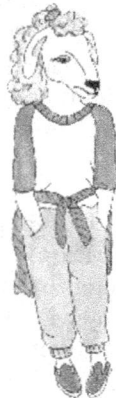

Figure 2.4 Sharla the Shameful Sheep

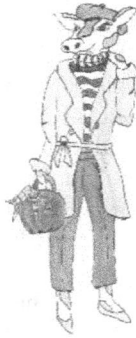

Figure 2.5 Contessa the Controlling Cow

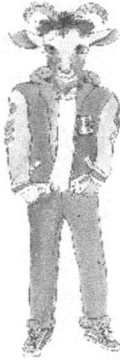

Figure 2.6 Eddie the Escape Goat

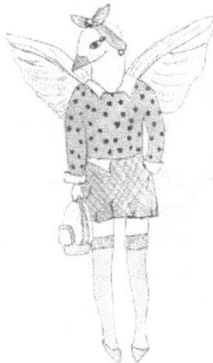

Figure 2.7 Shalom the Dove of Peace

Claire Controls

Claire was highly anxious. She presented with separation anxiety, and it was wreaking havoc on her family's life. Claire was now six and needing to go to school. Her Mom had been able to help in the kindergarten classroom, but now she had a new job on the other side of town. It was up to Claire to make it to and through the school day on her own. The family was now on a rigorous regimen working tirelessly not to upset Claire. The strict regimen was directed solely by Claire. However, this was not apparent yet to her or her family. They were in survival and unable to see that they were maneuvering under a six-year-old dictatorship. They walked on eggshells making sure not to upset Claire. If they did bother her, they relayed that "all hell would break loose." Claire would fall on the floor, grasping kitchen table legs as they tried to pick her up to carry her to their SUV for school. She would scream and cry and even passed out once.

Her fear was real, which was the difficult part as none of them wanted to see her suffering. She would scream out in pain, worried that her Mom and Dad would die or never come back if they left her. She couldn't sleep alone, eat alone. She had to leave the bathroom door open to freely dialogue back and forth with her Mom to make sure she was still there. They brought her into my office, all five of them looking a ghostly pallor with red-rimmed eyes. They let her know that she could choose to talk to me with the family there or alone. It probably goes without saying which option she picked.

When she refused to answer any of my questions in the session, they gave her the option of leaving ten minutes early if she answered. This satisfied her, and we started to talk. (I was quickly aware that this child was controlling her environment.) She was allowed all of the decision-making in the first session. Eventually, I would need to step in as a more authoritative role to disrupt the pattern of control and see where that might lead. There was not enough rapport yet built, and I also needed to, as Terry D. Hargrave says, "chase the pain" to see what lay behind the controlling coping. The following conversation began:

THERAPIST: So, Claire, can you tell me about what it is like for you when Mom wakes you up in the morning and says it is time for school?
CLAIRE: I get really scared. (Claire began to shake and cry.)
THERAPIST: It sounds like you get scared of what your Mom and Dad., and brother are saying. I wonder what we are afraid of?
(The therapist deciding to use bilateral movement to help calm midbrain anxiety, tossed a soft-ball to her, she caught it and held onto it, turning it around in her hand.)
THERAPIST: Do you mind throwing that back to me?
(Claire tossed it back, and the therapist returned it to her)
THERAPIST: Good catch. Hmmm . . . I wonder if we could throw it back and forth with opposite hands like this. I'll catch it with my left hand

and throw it with my right. (Noticing that her family looks somewhat dysregulated as well, tossed another ball to Dad) Why don't you and Gabe try this too while Claire and I do it?

THERAPIST: So, Claire, what are we scared of when we leave Mom?

CLAIRE: I can't tell you. I mean, I don't know.

THERAPIST: (continuing to toss the ball) Okay, you don't want to tell me yet. That's okay for now. So, what are some things that you like to do? What is your doll's name?

CLAIRE: My doll's name is Amy. She is so cute, isn't she?

THERAPIST: She is very, very cute. I love her curly red hair and green eyes. She looks a lot like you.

CLAIRE: Yes, she is my twin doll. That is why my grandma bought her for me.

THERAPIST: I really like her. She looks pretty smart to me, and it seems like you take good care of her. What do you guys talk about?

CLAIRE: We talk about lots of things.

THERAPIST: What is she like? Why do you like her?

CLAIRE: Well, she is super nice to people, and she loves her family. She is good at playing soccer, and she is a really, really good singer.

THERAPIST: Those are all wonderful things. Do you think she would sing for me?

CLAIRE: (smiling and then looking embarrassed) Well, she is shy about it.

THERAPIST: Okay, I get it. Maybe she could sing for me sometime, though. I like singing too. What is one of her favorite songs?

CLAIRE: Well, her favorite singer is Ariana Grande.

THERAPIST: Do you like her too?

CLAIRE: I love her. She is so pretty and nice, and I like to dance to her songs.

THERAPIST: Maybe next time we can play one of her songs and dance while talking about stuff. (Dancing with children also helps calm anxiety, especially when we employ a swaying, almost rocking motion from one foot to the other.) I also want to introduce you to some of my puppets. They are a little bit shy to talk in front of parents though and sometimes can talk better with just me and kids. I have an idea. I know you don't want your parents to leave, but do you want to see a way to make sure that your parents are available if we need them and still get the puppets to talk?

CLAIRE: (tearing up but nodding yes)

THERAPIST: Okay, well, I have this yarn here, and we can give Mom or Dad the end of the ball of yarn, and then you can hold the other end. They can walk clear out to the lobby, and if you pull on the yarn like this, they can pull back. That way we can be sure that they are there. "Let's see if it works. (The therapist stands up, handing parents the ball of yarn. "Okay, you can take this down the hall to the lobby, and when Claire pulls it, make sure to pull it back."

(parents smile broadly and take the yarn to the lobby)

THERAPIST: Okay, Claire. Let's see if it works.

(Claire yanks the yarn and receives three tugs back. She smiles and does it several times before settling back into the conversation.)

THERAPIST: (introduces the puppets) These are my friends. Aren't they cute? I really like them. They are good friends, but sometimes it is sad because they feel a lot of pain. They feel pain in their hearts and sometimes heads, stomachs, or backs when someone leaves them or treats them in a mean way. They don't want people to go, and sometimes they really disagree with what people do. Do you know what they always want to know?

CLAIRE: That their friends and family like them?

THERAPIST: Yes, I think they always want to know that. And mostly, they want to know that they are safe and loved. (Therapist observes Claire pulling on the string when mentioning that they don't want people to leave and that they want to be loved.)

CLAIRE: Can I see them?

THERAPIST: Yes, of course, you can! What should we have them do together?

CLAIRE: Let's have them go on a date to the movies

THERAPIST: (Chuckles) Okay, let's do it! (The therapist purposefully picks Contessa the Controlling Cow to exaggerate the control response and effect frustration in the patient)

(Speaking through Contessa, the Controlling Cow) Guess what? I am going on a date to the movies with Eddie the Escape Goat tonight.

CLAIRE: (Picking up Sharla, the shameful sheep, and speaking) Oh, that will be fun. Can I come?

THERAPIST: (through Contessa) Well, I guess you can come, but you can't sit with Eddie and me because I need to have him all to myself!

CLAIRE: (through Sharla) Well, we can all be friends and sit together.

THERAPIST: (through Contessa) No, it doesn't work that way because this is a date, and I am already planning on where we will sit. We will need to sit at the end of the aisle because he will need to buy me a lot of stuff like candy and soda and a pretzel, and we will be getting up a lot, and I need to go with him so we can walk together. We don't want to have to worry about you, Sharla, and we might leave early because I need to get my beauty rest.

CLAIRE: (through Sharla) Well, that isn't very nice. What if he doesn't want to go with you to buy you all of that stuff?

THERAPIST: (through Contessa) He will, or I will start crying a lot, and I might throw a big, huge fit!! I can moo soooo loud, and it will hurt everyone's ears.

CLAIRE: (through Sharla) Well, I won't like it if you throw a fit! Can't you just be happy with going to the movie with all of your friends?

THERAPIST: (through Contessa) I am getting sad just talking about this, Sharla. (starting to cry) I just want you and Brutus to sit in front of us where I can see you and make sure you don't leave. In case Eddie doesn't buy me candy, you can go with me and buy me some. I want you to sit three rows in front of us. Do you want me to write out instructions of where I want you to go?

CLAIRE: No. I do not want instructions! I want to sit where I want to sit. You are not a good friend!! You are so bossy! I think we should all decide where we want to sit and usually when you go to the movies you sit with your friends!

THERAPIST: (through Contessa) (in an angry voice) Well, I never!! I know what is best because I have been on four dates and you have not ever been on a date.

CLAIRE: How do you know? I have been on ten dates!

THERAPIST: Putting down puppet and bringing in Shalom the Dove of Peace to talk to them;

(through Shalom) Hi ladies! Oh, my goodness. It sounds like you are fighting. Oh, and sorry,

Claire, can you be Contessa now because I am Shalom?

CLAIRE: Okay, yes, I can be Contessa. (Claire picks up Contessa.)

THERAPIST: (through Shalom) What is wrong, Contessa? I can hear from way up in my nest in that very tall tree, and you sound very bossy. I heard you say you will throw a tantrum if you can't get candy with Eddie.

CLAIRE: (through Contessa) Yes. I need to go *everywhere* with Eddie.

THERAPIST: (through Shalom) What would it look like if you threw a tantrum? Would you throw things at the wall or scream and stop your feet?

CLAIRE: (through Contessa) No, I wouldn't do those things. I would probably just lay down and cry really hard and say. Don't leave me!!

THERAPIST: (through Shalom) I wonder why it would be so hard for you if Eddie left?

CLAIRE: (through Contessa) Because he can't leave me, I get really sad and worry about him.

THERAPIST: (through Shalom) Hmmm, I am so curious to know if you get more worried about yourself or Eddie?

CLAIRE: (through Contessa without hesitation) I am much more worried about him!

THERAPIST: (through Shalom) What are you worried about?

CLAIRE: (through Contessa) I am worried something horrible might happen to him and he might not come back, that maybe I would never see him again. Possibly there would be a tornado or a person with a gun, or a monster could get him.

THERAPIST: (through Shalom) Ahh, that must feel scary. What does that tell you about yourself, Contessa? What does it mean that Eddie could leave and not come back?

CLAIRE: (through Contessa) That's easy. It means I am scared all the time because people that I like aren't safe.

Are you safe?

CLAIRE: (through Contessa) I feel like I am safe, but people aren't safe when they aren't with me. I am very good at taking care of people.

We ended the session shortly after this. The therapist learned some vital things in this session and came up with a solid hypothesis about the patient's pain cycle. The therapist was able first to observe the family interaction. In this case, it was therapeutically helpful to ask the family to leave to establish some authority and disrupt the family's system of the child being in control. It was important to see experientially how this would play out.

Once alone with her, the therapist used the coping characters to explore further how and why control was used to cope with her pain. She was able to use the knowledge that control is nearly always indicative of a safety violation. Many therapists may be tempted to chase the controlling behaviors rather than the pain underneath. It is imperative to note how the control manifests as there is an element of behavioral therapy included in restoration therapy; however, this alone usually only produces second-order change. We need to find the primary emotion and painful feelings to help the client achieve first-order and lasting change.

We saw with this client that, somewhat surprisingly, she was not scared for her own well-being but rather for the well-being of her loved ones. Her sense of control gave her a false sense of security. When her family members were out of her "watchful care of them," She voiced that the world felt

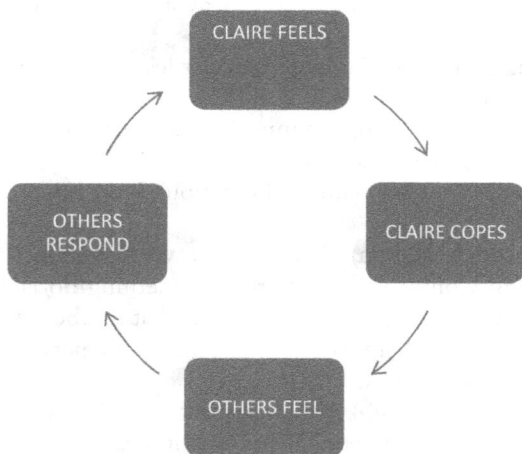

Figure 2.8 Claire's Pain Cycle

Claire's Pain Cycle Caption

"unsafe and scary" acting in controlling ways allowed her to feel a sort of momentary power rather than powerlessness. When she felt powerless, she sought to control circumstances by becoming dramatic, catastrophic and controlling.

It would help sketch out her pain cycle that would likely look something like the table below, although Claire's feelings and coping words would be different. The terms are different to provide helpful practice. Before moving to the next page, what are the three painful feeling words that Claire is likely experiencing? How does she specifically cope with these feelings? Please take a moment to figure out what they may be and sketch out her respective pain cycle.

Claire feels:

Unsafe
Out of Control
Powerless

Claire Copes by:

Catastrophizing
Controlling
Being Bossy

Likely, we will find that this is a pretty accurate depiction of Claire's pain cycle. When we are working with adults, it can often take longer to figure this process out. With children, it usually takes just a session or two. We hold the hypothesis of this pain cycle loosely, however, and remain open to it changing. It helps confirm or reorganize our hypothesis upon further investigative observation during play and some direct questioning. Kids, like adults, also become increasingly dysregulated during play when we hit upon and begin to act out the child's pain cycle rather than someone else's pain cycle. This is due to it "touching a nerve," so to speak, or a wound not entirely healed.

It is essential to use language like "we" instead of "you" even though we are still externalizing the work through the puppets. Children identify much more personally with toys than an adult. The therapist, in this case, was careful not to accuse the puppets or scold them too much. Kids are often quite willing to reprimand their own behaviors. The angst they show at specific actions vs. others gives us great insight into their pain cycle.

The therapist was able to move through the first two goals in this session by first defining the pain and second being able to identify the coping. In playing with Claire, it became evident by her bold nature that she likely had a fight response to pain. Due to her anxious behavior presentation, her particular fight response of coping through controlling behaviors rose from feeling unsafe. It is remarkable in working with children how quickly they can verbalize feeling unsafe and or unloved.

It is important to remember that control and blame are the fight responses stemming from feeling unsafe and unloved. The following is a scenario of another child who copes through blaming behaviors when he is in emotional pain. His father had called me and let me know that his five-year-old son was getting in trouble at home and kindergarten. His parents were experiencing an "in-home separation." They had moved to different bedrooms and rarely spoke to each other. He said the kids were unaware of their emotional separation and seemed to think everything was normal as they never mentioned it. I let Dad know that it would be ideal if they could both bring him to the appointment together so that we could talk over the signed paperwork and help their child be more comfortable. He answered that they could not be in the same room together, and this is what they both were afraid of. Was there anyway just one of them could bring him to see? Otherwise, it wouldn't work. He explained this in an agitated manner. He went on to say that none of this was his fault, and his wife had become so negative in their interactions they could no longer work together. He wondered aloud angrily why family therapists seemed to be so hard to work with. This was his third call to find a fit for their family. I could hear in his voice that he would not bend on joining his wife in session. I pushed a bit more, remarking that it is really best to have both parents come if they can do so, but I also understood that sometimes this might be too difficult. I did say I needed one of them to go and that both would need to sign the paperwork (as it appeared divorce and a custody battle was quite likely.)

Identifying the Fight Response in Parents and the Threat of Legality in Work with Kids

Sadly, the threat of legality is one of the primary reasons why many clinicians refuse to work with children. This is entirely plausible as the risks of being asked to go to court are higher. However, we can do much and say before the beginning of therapy to avoid being summoned to court. Because court involvement scares so many clinicians away from helping kids, it is worth spending a bit of time addressing the issue.

It seems most often, parents who cope with the fight response end up in court and are significantly more likely to subpoena the therapist or the records. As we learn more about Restoration Therapy and identify various coping methods, it becomes easier to ascertain in the first phone call or meeting if parents react with a fight response. If this is the case, we proceed even more cautiously to cover our bases regarding court involvement before beginning therapy.

I always explain to parents if I hear a hint of divorce or current custody battle is that "I find it very important therapeutically for kids to have a safe space to talk about their feelings. They invariably feel caught in the middle and do not have a place to talk about their pain. I tell parents that

I must be allowed to provide a safe space, and I want to honor their child's confidentiality. I explain that so often, kids are worried that a parent may get mad at them. I further educate them that it is essential to their child's progress that they feel free from punishment when expressing a feeling. I let parents know that no one should ever be punished for having a feeling, and during divorce, as the parents are well aware, there are lots of painful and hurtful emotions flying around. I follow this explanation with the options of therapeutic interventionists and mediators who work with the court. I let them know that our ethical standard as Licensed Marriage and Family Therapists restrict us from making any recommendation about parenting or custody arrangements. If this is what they are looking for, I understand. However, I let them know I am not the right person for that particular job.

I am careful to provide a safe space for their children to talk through their emotions and will keep their confidentiality unless it is a safety issue. I invite parents to join whenever they want a broad update on their child's progress or possible tips on parenting or co-parenting. I remind them I will not disclose details of what the kids are saying to me unless I have the child's permission. I then give parents a way out by saying that they can think about it and call me back if they would like. It is essential to exercise caution and not coerce anyone into a type of therapy that they are not desiring.

If a parent decides to allow their child to enter therapy with me, I am careful to repeat these ethical practices in front of the child, reiterating what I do and do not need to share with parents or an adult guardian. Often this proves to be rapport building as we brainstorm together. I ask questions like, "So if a kid tells me that they played on their iPad past the time they were supposed to be asleep in bed, would I have to say something?" Or, "If a kid told me that they were crying when they heard their parents fighting, would I have to say something?" Or, "I also have had kids say they wanted to spend more time at one house than the other; would I have to say something?" I follow with, what if a kid was being hurt by something or someone in their house, like beat up? Would I need to say something?"

I find it therapeutically and ethically appropriate to give children some power in their care. I am not interested in trapping them inadvertently into telling me something they are not ready to talk about yet. It is typically relatively easy to determine if a child is in danger, and if this is the case, of course, I readily advocate to remove them from any danger. I asked a colleague what one of her favorite things is about working with children, and she said it is the ability to provide a safe place for them and the relief that she sees when they finally trust that this is true.

After these initial conversations, it is beneficial to let children know that they can choose to talk about whatever they would like regarding what is said or what we do in counseling. I tell them that it will likely be helpful to communicate with their parents. Also, I let them know "it would be weird, and not okay, for any adult to ask a kid not to tell their parents something." They usually agree whole-heartedly with this. I remind them that they can talk about anything, but I can't. This is part of my job to protect what they tell me, and I hope they can learn to feel safe.

Discussions like these invariably provide buy-in from parents, as it seems intuitive to them that their kids need a place to let things out. If they still desire court intervention at this point, they may opt-out of the therapeutic relationship with me, and that is okay too. Doing our due diligence and explaining why our job is not conducive to working with the courts is very helpful. I may be fortunate, but I have never been called into court. I work with children and divorce consistently.

Interestingly, people who often want to take a therapist into court tend to deal with their pain through blame or control. If we see this as a tendency, it is wise to cover everything with cautious clarity from the initial call and assessment. Often when children trend toward blame or control, they likely have a parent who exhibits this as well. Blame and control are no worse for relationships than any of the other maladaptive coping methods. However, it can lead to court proceedings. Sometimes court is necessary, and I remain grateful for our justice system. Court involvement does create extra work and stress for therapists and is usually the number one reason people avoid working with children. This is an unfortunate reality; however, in implementing wisdom in our initial conversation, court involvement is most often prevented when it isn't needed or desired.

Brody Blames

The young man we are about to meet was quite responsive to my letting him know that he had a safe place to vent in front of his Dad. He smiled, looking shyly at me and back to his father. I asked his Dad if he and his Mom were okay with Brody, saying whatever he wanted about his feelings in my office. His Dad said yes and that he would let Brody decide what to or not talk about regarding how his time with Ms. Nancy went. I excused Dad to the lobby and Brody, and I got to work trying to figure out what these sour painful feelings were that were tempting him to act out at home and in school.

The reader is invited to take some notes while observing the following vignette. It is helpful to try and ascertain what Brody's painful emotions maybe and then how he copes with each painful feeling:

Brody Blames

Session 1

THERAPIST: (smiling) Alright, Brody, how about we sit on the floor? The therapist moves the table to create more floor space in the room. So, can you tell me what your week has been like?

BRODY: Um . . . Pretty good. (Pointing to the toy bin of matchbox cars) Can we play with these cars now?

THERAPIST: Hmm . . . Cars are really fun to play with, huh? Maybe we can play with them for a little bit. First, I want you to meet some of my friends (gathering the puppets Therapist begins to introduce them). This is Brutus, the Blaming badger, and when he gets upset, he likes to blame other people. Do you know what that means?

BRODY: Yes, that means he tells other people it is their fault or that they did something wrong.

THERAPIST: Oh, my goodness! You are exactly right; that is just what he does! Now let's guess the next one. This is Sharla, the Shameful Sheep. This one might be harder to guess. When she gets upset, or there is a disagreement or argument, she shames herself. What do we think that word shame might look like?

BRODY: Oh, maybe she puts her head down and cries?

THERAPIST: Yes, exactly! She does that a lot, and sometimes I wonder why?

BRODY: Maybe because she thinks no one likes her anymore, and she feels stupid.

THERAPIST: Yes, Brody! When we shame ourself we feel like no one likes us and like maybe we can't do anything right, and we are a bad person or sheep.

BRODY: I felt that way before.

THERAPIST: Yes, most of us have felt that way at some point. When did you feel that way?

BRODY: I felt that way when my Mom and Dad said I had to come to a counselor. Because only I had to come. They think my sister is the good kid, and I am the bad kid.

THERAPIST: Oh, I hear what you are saying. Unfortunately, many kids and even big people feel that way when they go to a counselor. I wish we didn't have to feel ashamed about it. There are a lot of really, really good reasons to go to a counselor. Are you feeling like Sharla right now?

BRODY: No. This is a lot different than I thought it would be. I thought you would be sitting in a big tall chair like a lifeguard has and have a megaphone, and maybe you would be yelling out questions at me like, "What is wrong with you? Why are you such a bad kid?" I thought you would have the only chair, and I would have to stand up the whole time, and you would yell at me like this (pointing his finger at the floor and pretending to yell.) I felt a lot better when I saw that you are at this house place and that you just live here in this living room and have soft couches and lamps and toys. I don't see your TV and bed, where are they?

THERAPIST: (smiling) This does look like a living room, but it is my office. I have a house somewhere else.

BRODY: (looking around) Oh. I like it here, and I like that you aren't yelling at me.

THERAPIST: I can promise I won't ever yell at you.

BRODY: Thanks. (Pointing back to the puppets) What is that cow's name?

THERAPIST: This is Contessa, the Controlling Cow, and she likes to control everything and is pretty bossy.

BRODY: Like my Mom.

THERAPIST: Well, I'm not sure. Do you think your Mom is bossy?

BRODY: She is sooo bossy. She yells at me and says, "why don't you ever listen to me?" Your sisters listen to me, and they stay out of trouble.

THERAPIST: Hmmm . . . Yes, Moms sometimes say things like that. I wonder how that makes you feel?

BRODY: It makes me mad, and then I say things that get me in big trouble!

THERAPIST: Like, what kind of things do we say?

BRODY: I just tell her she doesn't know everything, and it isn't my fault for not hanging my jacket up because my sister Betsy threw it on the ground. Even if she really didn't throw it on the ground, I say that because I am so mad!

THERAPIST: Then, what happens?

BRODY: Then I get a time out, and sometimes I get Tabasco on my tongue because I lied.

THERAPIST: Oh, dear. I bet that doesn't taste good.

BRODY: Nope, but I don't cry about it. I'm not a dumb baby. (takes the badger and hits the sheep across the room, now picking up the goat.) What is this goat's name?

THERAPIST: Oh wow, Brutus is mad at Sharla. I can see that, and the goat is named Eddie. Eddie the Escape Goat.

BRODY: Eddie the Escape Goat? What does he do?

THERAPIST: Well, when he is upset or feels like someone is upset with him, he runs away. Sometimes he plays a lot of video games and puts his headphones on so he can't hear things that he doesn't want to hear. He hates fighting!

BRODY: (Grabs Eddie and runs with him around the room, hiding him in a corner.)

THERAPIST: (Laughs), exactly!!

Now, let's listen to a song about these puppets to get to know them a little better and do a puppet show (plays song, while the song is playing the therapist invites the child to act out words of the song collaboratively, creating a puppet show.)

Coping Characters Song Lyrics

I'm here to tell a story about my friends from the farm down the way.

Now, if you listen closely, I know that we, we can learn something today.

It starts off with Brutus the Badger. He likes to point fingers even though it doesn't matter; he says, "It was not me. It was you, can't you see that this is true?"

He says, "I'm not wrong; I did no harm; it was someone else at the farm.

I didn't, I didn't start the fight. I didn't start the fight!"
In comes Sharla, saying, "Maybe Brutus was right,
I'm the one to blame. I didn't play by the rules of the game.
It's all my fault. I can't stand tall.
I feel so bad inside; I cannot hide; I wanna cry.
I'm the one to blame; I feel like I ruined everybody's day."
Oh, lookout. Here comes Contessa! She's saying, "Get out of my
    way."
She says, "Listen up to me, and hear what I have to say.
Now everyone needs to pay attention to me.
Can't you see that all of you are wrong except for me?
Don't' say a word and focus on me.
If you think you can fix your own problems if you think you're the
    one that can solve them. I'm here to say that that is not true,
Because you're not me, and you are you!"
Meanwhile, everybody wonders where Eddie has gone this time?
He likes to run away whenever there is a fight.
He's gone again, gone like the wind; he ran away right when the
    drama came, just like the other day,
Now he's hiding in a stack of hay
with his hoofs over his ears, he's hoping that the fighting disappears
There are many ways to deal with the problems that you have. But
    I can promise, these are not good ways to react.
Maybe start off with a hug and add a little love; say sorry when you
    can helping hand in hand.
So start off with a hug and add a little love; say sorry when you can
    helping hand in hand.
So start off with a hug and add a little love.

(Music and Lyrics by Micah John Frigaard, 2019)

BRODY: (smiling) These puppets are funny. We did a good job! Can we
    show my Mom and Dad this puppet show?
THERAPIST: Yes, we certainly can if you would like to. I think that is a
    wonderful idea! You did a really good job. So now that we know what
    these puppets act like when they are upset, which one do you think you
    might be most like?
BRODY: Shyly points to Brutus and then picks him up.
THERAPIST: Ahhh . . . Mmm, so when we get upset, we sometimes blame
    people, get mad and say it is their fault?
BRODY: Yep! And then I get in big trouble!
THERAPIST: Yes, Brutus gets in trouble for that a lot too. He isn't always like
    that, though. Sometimes he is different.
BRODY: Just like me! A lot of times, I am different.
THERAPIST: I know you are. What is usually happening when you are
    different?

BRODY: Like when it is my birthday party, I am so nice to people because everyone is singing to me and looking at me and I like it.

THERAPIST: Does it feel good when people are paying attention to you and celebrating you.

BRODY: vigorously nods his head, yes. (smiling.)

THERAPIST: What happens when people ignore us?

BRODY: I get angry

THERAPIST: Where do you feel the anger in your body.

BRODY: In my fists and teeth and my eyes squint.

THERAPIST: Like this? (visually acts out clenching teeth and fists and narrowing eyes)

BRODY: Yes, exactly, only my eyes are more open than yours are.

THERAPIST: (smiles) Thank you so much for helping me understand what it looks and feels like. You said your Mom could be like Contessa? What about Dad? Which one might he act like?

BRODY: I think he acts like Brutus too. Hey! That is probably why my Mom says, and you are just like your Dad., only a littler one.

THERAPIST: laughs.

BRODY: Oh! and my older sister, Becky, is just like Eddie the Escape Goat; she puts her earphones in and plays video games all of the time. When everyone else is yelling, I just scream louder when she does this because she doesn't pay attention to anything I do. It makes me so mad!! We have fun together when she lets me play with her toys. I don't know which one my little sister is like. She is only two.

THERAPIST: Yes, we all act like these puppets sometimes when we get upset, and usually we act more like one or two than the others. What do you think about asking your family next time, whoever brings you, and we could see which animals they think they act like when they are upset?

BRODY: Oh yeah! Let's do that, and I know that I am right, though!!

THERAPIST: You have done a really great job thinking about what these puppets are like.

BRODY: (smiles) Thank you!

THERAPIST: So now before we have to go, let see what we remember. Do you think you can pick up each puppet and tell me their name and what they act like?

BRODY: Yes!! Okay, this is Brutus the Badger, and he is kind of like me. He mostly blames other people and argues when he is mad, or if people are mean to him, or if he feels like no one likes him. This is Contessa, the Controlling cow, and she is soooo bossy, and she tells other people what to do and makes a lot of plans. She gets mad at people when they don't do what she says. This is Sharla, the shameful sheep. She feels really sad when people argue with her and thinks she is a very bad sheep, and this is Eddie the Escape Goat (runs around the room with Eddie giggling. The therapist joins the child running after him around the coffee table.)

THERAPIST: And what does Eddie do when something is upsetting?

BRODY: He puts his headphones on and runs away and just leaves.

THERAPIST: Wow! That is just super how quickly you got to know these guys.

BRODY: (grinning) I know I am really smart.

THERAPIST: I can tell! Okay, let's put these things away and move our table back. Do you think you are strong enough to help me do that?

BRODY: I am so strong. (showing his muscles)

THERAPIST: I thought so. (Putting toys away and walking him out to the lobby.)

This case study is another example of the therapist moving through the first objective's two elements, identifying and understanding the pain cycle. Brody, like Claire, has a fight instinct, but instead of being controlling, he copes through blame and anger. We explored what his blaming and anger look like and were able to observe it in action. In upcoming sessions, we would likely intervene by using Shalom the Dove of Peace to talk over any violent action occurring between the coping characters, like when Brutus the Blaming Badger threw Sharla across the room. We could then play out the relational consequences. For example, Sharla would have likely shamed herself and possibly shut down. The child could work through this experientially through play and would likely become dysregulated. When this occurred, the therapist could introduce Shalom, the Dove of Peace, who could start challenging the painful feelings with the truth of the child's identity. In so doing, we could start moving to the second objective, which is endeavoring to help the child identify the emotionally regulating message of truth.

Practice

What has the therapist learned about Brody's pain cycle? Please attempt to guess his top three painful feelings and correlated coping responses.

Fill in the blanks here with your best guess before turning the page:

Brody feels:

1.
2.
3.

Brody copes

1.
2.
3.

Answers

Brody feels

1. Unloved
2. Disconnected
3. Insignificant

Brody copes

1. Blaming
2. Acting out
3. Angry

You may have filled in synonyms to these feelings and ways of coping or the exact words. As we meet more often with the client, we will be engaged in proving or disproving these preliminary hypotheses. It is also imperative to work on emotional vocabulary with our pediatric clients. The lack of being able to articulate precisely is another reason why many clinicians are hesitant to work with children as their vocabulary is underdeveloped. This lack of vocabulary is why working with children in their language of play is so helpful. However, we can find even greater success by teaching kids emotional vocabulary words in poignant and memorable ways. We can do this by creating scenarios in the room where we act out through puppets or other toys what various emotions look and sound like. Also, we can explore which types of conflicts typically ignite particular emotions. There are significant differences between feeling words like nervous or terrified, or behavioral, coping, words such as catastrophic or grumpy. As kids learn vocabulary and experience their emotions in action, their ability to pinpoint their feelings and responses allows them first to validate their painful feeling, regulate, and then change their responses. Words are typically the first way children start to employ and understand the use of symbolism. They also use toys to symbolize meaning as well (Myers & Dewall, 2010).

   The following chart can be helpful for both the clinician and the client to practice and identify vocabulary words pertaining to the Pain and Coping cycle:

Painful Feelings			
Unloved		**Unsafe**	
Unloved	Inadequate	Powerless	Vulnerable
Unworthy	Unacceptable	Out of Control	Invalidated
Insignificant	Hopeless	Unsafe	Failure
Alone	Unwanted	Insecure	
Worthless	Disconnected	Devalued	
Unknown	Defective	Not measuring up	

Figure 2.9 Painful Feelings and Coping Responses

COPING

BLAME	SHAME	CONTROL	ESCAPE
Blame others	Depressed	Perfectionistic	Drugs/Alcohol
Rage	Negative	Defensive	Numb out
Angry	Anxious	Judging	Impulsive
Sarcastic	Inconsolable	Demanding	Video games
Arrogant	Catastrophizing	Critical	Avoid issues
Aggressive	Whine/Needy	Nagging	Hide information
Discouraging	Manipulates	Lecture	Get dramatic
Threatening	Withdraw to pout	Withdraw to defend	Act selfish
Hold grudges	Isolate	Intellectualize	Minimizes
Retaliatory	Fault finding	Controlling	Withdraw to avoid
Withdraw to punish	Shame self		Irresponsible
Disrespectful			Escape

Figure 2.9 (Continued)

Stage	Age range	What happens at this stage?
Sensorimotor	0–2 years old	Coordination of senses with motor responses, sensory curiosity about the world. Language used for demands and cataloguing. Object permanence is developed.
Preoperational	2–7 years old	Symbolic Thinking, use of proper syntax and grammar to express concepts. Imagination and intuition are strong, but complex abstract thoughts are still difficult. Conservation is developed.
Concrete Operational	7–11 years old	Concepts attached to concrete situations. Time, space, and quantity are understood and can be applied, but not as independent concepts.
Formal Operational	11 years and older	Theoretical, hypothetical, and counterfactual thinking. Abstract logic and reasoning. Strategy and planning become possible. Concepts learned in one context can be applied in another.

Figure 2.10 Piaget's stages of Cognitive development

Through developing greater vocabulary, Piaget's stages of development can likely be moved through more quickly. A child's use of symbolism begins in the Preoperational stage and develops into the ability to move into the Concrete Operational stage. These stages, as Piaget agreed, are somewhat fluid. If a child is still very much in the Preoperational stage, there is still much great work done through play. It helps identify what stage of development a child is in to work with them most effectively (Myers & Dewall, 2010).

It can be viewed as a blessing that kids are working from an egocentric place in therapy and still displaying animism characteristics (the belief that toys have feelings and a voice). As they give animals or toys this voice, we can almost be certain that the animals' words and feelings are their own. This makes the child's own emotions quite transparent to the observing therapist, which allows us to understand their pain. As we did with Claire, I so often witness that their dolls or superheroes are their emotional twins. When we ask these twins questions, we get the child's personal answers. When we care for the toy, we care for them. Also, kids can tell us very clearly what they need in this way.

One of my colleagues, who is currently employing Restoration Play Therapy in his work with children, told me the following story last week. His daughter, whom I like to call "Baby Mary," is just now two years old. She is wonderfully winsome and fearless. She has been in the healthy bio-psychosocial habit of snacking and soothing by breastfeeding before bed-time. Michael and his wife decided it was time to wean her just after her second birthday entirely. I am sure that the disruption in her comforting schedule seemed an entirely unacceptable birthday present to her. This new change was met with frustration and distress.

My colleague and his wife patiently spoke tenderly to her, explaining that she was a big girl now, and she would be just fine going to bed without her soothing snack. They offered her cuddly stuffed animals, extra reading time, and alternative physical affection.

Their valiant conscientious efforts to convince her all would be well only fell on deaf and hurting ears. Michael, my colleague, had the idea of using her language of play to try and get their point across. As he moved to tuck her in, he picked up a little stuffed dog that she was cuddling with and started speaking through it.

DOG: Hi, Mary. I want to nurse tonight, but they say I can't. (pretending to cry) I don't know what to do.

MARY: (reaching out to pat him) It's okay, dog. You can do it. You are a big girl now. You have this pacifier. (putting the pacifier in the dog's mouth, covering it with a blanket, and kissing it.)

DOG: But I still really want to. It makes me so sad and lonely.

MARY: You okay, Dog. I will help you. You are big, and you can do it.

Michael observed the interaction and watched how Baby Mary showed them what she needed. She needed affection, support and encouragement, and a little help. She was also able to process emotion and how to regulate (self-soothe) through play. She and her Dad both were able to collabora-tively engage in a verbal and physical demonstration of creating an accept-able alternative. Michael said it was amazing how she was able to hold the dog and go right to sleep without further tears.

Playing is imperative, and sometimes directive play is essential as it provides context for the child's pain and gives them a choice within certain parameters.

Michael didn't dictate how the story would end, but he started it off in the right setting. If he would have set, upset Mary down in a room and simply asked her to "start playing." He may have gotten somewhere, but it is hard to tell if the play would have been pertinent to the specific matter at hand.

Children have varied personalities like adults. It would be poor judgment to assume that they are the same or even similar. Just as we adapt our therapeutic methodology for adults, we must do it for children as well. I know of therapists who use dance and native drum beat music while water coloring with their clients, and depending on the client, it can be wildly successful. Imagine, however, a typical "type A" engineer with a shirt and tie entering this same environment. It would likely be very uncomfortable for him. I can envision him pulling at his collar nervously and feeling very out of place. Kids are wired similarly. In my combined experience of teaching then working with kids in the psychology field for nearly 20 years, I have seen this be true. Some kids can work well in a less linear environment, but many become quite distressed without explicit instruction. It seems these kids have been largely ignored. Kids who have a blended personality of boldness and creativity may do well with a non-directive approach. However, we must not overlook other personality types.

Most of the books out there and workshops on play therapy are very non-directive. As I have practiced this approach, I have witnessed overwhelm set in. For instance, one respected intervention is the kinetic drawing, where the therapist instructs the child to draw each member of their family doing something. Although somewhat directive, I have seen one of two responses over and again. One child will grab the markers using a variety of colors and get to work. They can come up with reasonably impressive drawings and then take off explaining their family to me in animated terms. Others will stall and fearfully tell me that they can't draw and, if they are brave enough, will ask me for further instruction. When I answer with the favored non-directive approach, which is: "do whatever you want, there is no right or wrong." Some kids visibly cringe and often ask me if I can draw it for them or what colors to use etc. . . . We may infer that these kids are traumatized, timid, scared, afraid to take risks, or perfectionists. Perhaps this is true; however, our goal of finding out about their family has not been accomplished. Creative kids often feel stifled by too many rules. Rule followers feel equally stifled by unclear expectations. Desiring explicit instruction is neither pathological nor unhealthy; it is personality preference. Once again, art without science and science without art results in a cheapened outcome. Creativity within a structure is where the best sort of beauty is discovered. RT for kids has an adapted version of a Kinetic drawing specific to identifying the pain and peace cycle. This is further explained in part two of the book.

Summary

The current research shows that emotional pain from relational conflict triggers our amygdala and sends our nervous system into a fight or flight response (Hanna, 2014). This chapter focused on the fight responses rather than the flight responses. As a marriage and family therapist, a primary task is to help our clients find relief from the pain of discordant or conflictual relationships. When working with children, it is constructive first to identify destructive behaviors stemming from blame, shame, control, or escape. Armed with this knowledge and a willingness to play through various conflictual scenarios with a child, we can observe and ask good questions, which leads to a discovery of the sore emotions that live underneath the coping. When we have a firm grasp and understanding of these painful feelings ultimately stemming from feeling unloved or unsafe, we can begin to tie each form of coping to the specific pain. When we have completed this task, we then help the child recognize their pain cycle. This leads us to the next step of beginning to look at the peace cycle.

References

Bowlby, J. (1988). *A secure base.* Basic Books.

Feight, R. (2021). *Coping characters.*

Frigaard, M. (2019). *Pain to peace song.*

Hanna, S. M. (2014). *The transparent brain in couple and family therapy: Mindful integrations with neuroscience.* Routledge.

Hargrave, T. D. (2019). *Advances and techniques in restoration therapy.* Routledge and Taylor & Francis Group.

MacLean, P. D. (1990). *The triune brain in evolution: Role in paleo cerebral functions.* Springer.

Myers, D. G., & DeWall, C. N. (2010). *Exploring psychology.* Worth Publishers.

3 Fight or Flight? Let's Take Flight

Rather than fighting during a threat, many children tend to take flight in an attempt to flee the emotional pain of feeling unloved or unsafe. Like fighting, this effort may work momentarily but does not solve the problem and will only exacerbate the intensity of these painful core emotions over time. Children take flight through shaming themselves or by using various methods of escape. When a love violation threatens a secure attachment, children tend to disappear into shame. When their safety is threatened, they find a way to escape. These ways of coping are intuitive and understandable (Hargrave, 2019). It is helpful for the therapist to identify the coping and work backward to the pain behind it. Behind the shame and escaping, the therapist can discover the wounds in need of healing. The following vignettes, including therapist intervention, will prove helpful when working with children who instinctively move toward a flight response.

It slowly sunk in as she watched popular Juniper Joy passing out invitations. She was not invited to the fifth-grade class party; she put her head down on the desk and let the tears come. Why didn't anyone like her? Perhaps, she wasn't as pretty as the other girls. They had nice clothes and hair; hers was too curly. She was scrawny and had no figure. She probably was never going to have one. None of the boys liked her, and she said stupid things. That is why she was unwelcome. Her friend noticed her crying and passed her a note; she imagined it said something hateful and didn't bother to look at it. When the bell rang, she knew everyone was thinking about how ugly and worthless she was. She was so steeped in shame that she couldn't see straight. She ran shins first into the busses metal stairs. She winced at the pain, but it was nothing like the pain she felt inside. The Lying Lizard was shouting at her. "You are worthless; you are unloved, you are stupid." Instead of fighting, she shrunk inward, almost disappearing.

Shame and escape are examples of answering the poisoned words of the Lying Lizard through the flight response. As therapists, it can be common to have greater compassion for those responding with the flight response, as they can be easier to get along with and may even appear more vulnerable. The first may be accurate but not necessarily the latter. Our compassion

DOI: 10.4324/9781003025504-3

ought to be equal for the fight and flight response because when the Lying Lizard screams at these children, the pain is equal.

After the pain, the coping ignites like a match to gasoline, and children become quickly dysregulated. The path through the pain into peace is the same with the flight responder but uses different words. As you read the following cases, start to employ what you have learned so far as we complete the first two elements of the first objective in Restoration Therapy, identifying the pain and how they are coping with that pain (Hargrave, 2019). After this chapter, we will discover how to accomplish the final three objectives, which allow our clients to move from pain to peace.

Stewart and Shame

Early on in my work with kids, I scheduled an appointment for a little boy named Stewart. Still hesitant about working with children, I mentally prepared to meet him in the lobby, I took a deep breath, said a prayer, and opened the door. I instantly was moved by his look of sweet innocence mixed with some trepidation. At his Dad's bidding, he rose from his seat when I entered the waiting room. He was peering up at me, jet black hair and big green eyes behind thick, black-rimmed glasses. I knew from the initial phone interview that he was six years old and that Mom had recently abandoned the family due to drug addiction. I had heard he was having trouble sleeping and could not go to school some days due to intense anxiety and panic attacks.

I thought he was absolutely adorable. At the time, I wasn't sure if it was unprofessional to think of a little patient as absolutely adorable; regardless, I did. He reached out tentatively to shake my hand, and as I placed my hand in his small one, I knew instinctively that I wanted to do this again and again. It is an honor to hold many little hands and walk with kids through their painful and unfair journeys. In this sacred territory, we are privileged to empower, educate, and equip children while arming them with the truth about their unique wonderful selves. As therapists, we want to help kids feel safe and learn how to discern safe from unsafe relationships. We want them to feel significant and loved. We *want* much for our little clients, and we also know we *need* to do all of the above with excellence. I continue to be driven to find a way to help children, some of the most powerless among us, systematically and creatively. Restoration Therapy is a tangible theory to help provide direction in providing the best sort of therapy to children.

This young man and I quickly built great rapport; while playing with matchbox cars in session and creating parking spaces in lots constructed from yellow pencils, he shared his fears with me. He taught me how to parallel park Big-Rigs with trailers without jack-knifing them. He was by far the better and more practiced of the two of us. He patiently explained spatial realities, angles, and how movement differs in reverse. Something I admittedly struggle with in real life. During this rapport-building exercise,

I was struck by the humanness of little people. They have unique interests and abilities. They respond to encouragement and discouragement in similar ways.

As I encouraged him, he got physically closer to me. Pretty soon, he was next to me on the floor, leaning into me so fully that it became hard for me to back my matchbox semi-truck around the corner into the driveway we had made. His head was against my shoulder, and he was rubbing my arm. I allowed him to be close and continued to play. I wasn't sure if this was appropriate professionally, but at the same time, I knew it would be inappropriately hurtful to pull away from him. Curious, I asked, "Who else do you like to cuddle with?" I allowed the question to hang while moving my truck backward and jack-knifing it again. I let out a defeated sigh, and He giggled.

"I used to cuddle with my Mom at night. I could hear her heartbeat. Sometimes I would be afraid that she would leave if I fell asleep. If her heartbeat was calm, I knew she would stay." He paused and looked up at me. Is your heartbeat slow or fast right now? He asked. "Slow," I replied, and his little mouth curved into a grin. "I wonder if you can remember what you felt like when she was holding you?" I ventured. His response took a few moments, and I watched his eyes move down and to the left, "I felt really good. Good and safe." He said and sighed. "What does good feel like?" I questioned. "Good feels like my tummy is warm and like everyone loves me." He hugged my arm closer as he said this, and I reached over and tousled his hair. It looks like it is time to start putting away our toys. We quietly moved to put them away, both reflective. I reflected that these precious little clients had the same core emotions as my adult clients. I was guessing their coping styles were the same as well.

Stewart is the boy who first started driving me to become a better child therapist and his words about how he felt with his Mom when she held him. He said he felt good and safe and explained that good meant loved. I was already learning the ins and outs of Restoration Therapy, and it instantly got me to thinking that if love and trustworthiness are the pillars of a healthy relationship. If our core needs are to feel loved and safe to form a healthy attachment, it was imperative to start working from this framework with kids and adults alike. When I began employing Restoration Therapy techniques with children, I thought it was common practice. I assumed that Restoration Therapy was applied to work with children around the world. Perhaps due to my teaching background and growing up in a family that valued and esteemed children, it made sense to me about how to adapt the theory. It came instinctively. I witnessed understanding by children and change in a more significant measure when using Restoration Therapy methods.

I had tried using other theories, including non-directive play therapy approaches. All of them felt uncomfortable; they were too nebulous. Although I have a very flexible nature, I had grown accustomed to working with objectives as a teacher. Treatment plans include objectives and goals, and I consistently felt confused about writing a treatment plan without knowing what steps I would use to reach the objective. When I began to move through the four goals of Restoration Therapy, my treatment plans made sense, and I finally had a way to measure progress. I knew when and where the client was getting stuck. I moved quickly through what they understood and knew when to slow down if they didn't quite have a handle on certain elements. After putting RT into practice, patient progress was more evident, and change was not only quicker but deeper. I experienced children finding lasting relief and behavioral changes. I started getting calls from churches and schools to work specifically with kids.

I learned a lot from Stewart about Restoration Therapy. He and I learned and flourished together in the model. I have many incredible memories of watching the power of the Restoration Therapy model at work. The following is one I won't soon forget.

STEWART: Ms. Nancy?

THERAPIST: Yes, Stewart.

STEWART: I was extra sad this week. I missed my Mom a lot, and I couldn't fall asleep.

THERAPIST: I imagine you do miss your Mom. What were you thinking about when you were trying to fall asleep?

STEWART: I was thinking about my video games and music.

THERAPIST: hmmm. Do you have a favorite song this week? (I had found Stewart usually had a favorite song, and it more often than not led us into his deeper emotions. It is uncanny how kids trend toward emotional health and find ways to soothe and express their sorrows. For some, it is drawing; for others, it is playing sports. For Stewart, it was trucks, engines of any kind, and music. As a children's therapist, it is essential to welcome the child's various forms of expression. It provides us with often incredible insight into their pain.)

STEWART: Yes, can we listen to "Hey Ho" by The Lumineers

THERAPIST: Yes, we can. Let me look it up.

I was vaguely familiar with the song as it had a catchy tune, but I had never taken the time to listen to the lyrics. I knew it was a love song.

We sat on separate couches as the song began. I typically searched YouTube for a version that showed the lyrics so that we could sing along together. Right after the introductory music was over and the words began, chills ran through me, and I struggled to fight back the tears as this song, discovered by a six-year-old, gave voice to his heart cry. For him, someone had written and performed a song that perfectly fit his feelings about his Mom abandoning his family and his sense of shame that led to his perfectionistic coping.

I struggled to sing as compassionate tears welled up within me, along with a sense of awe that a child figured out, and robustly embraced the healing qualities of music and lyrics. He did not notice my response, and perhaps, I am thankful. Although, there are appropriate times for clients to see our tears. He was sitting sideways on the small couch in my office, his feet up, eyes closed, and hugging a soft pillow. He was wholly lost in the song. I observed him singing every last word with a heartfelt expression, getting louder and louder, his face at times twisting in pain as the song progressed. I listened carefully, awestruck, while he grieved and sang about family, bleeding, sleeping alone, and the tearing separation from his Mom, whom he referred to as his "sweetheart."

THERAPIST: (after the song was over) Wow, Stewart. That is a perfect song. I am so glad that you asked me to play it.

STEWART: Yes, I really like it. It is sad.

THERAPIST: It is sad and good too. You did such a great job singing it. I wonder who you think about when you are singing it?

STEWART: My Mom. I think about her in my bed, and I keep saying I am so so so sorry. I don't know what I did to make you leave. I won't do it anymore. I just don't know what it was. I know I did something horrible, but I can't think of it. (starts to cry)

THERAPIST: (Moving over to sit next to him and allowing him some time to cry) Oh, Stewart. Can I tell you something that I know for sure?

STEWART: (sniffling) Yes.

THERAPIST: Almost every kid who comes to visit me with a Mom or Dad who leaves thinks that they did something horrible that made their parent go. But can I tell you something? Are you able to listen now, because I can wait until you feel ready? It's really important for you to hear this.

STEWART: Okay (cries some more) I feel really sad for those other kids. Do they know what they did wrong?

THERAPIST: (Moving closer to Stewart) Well, I want to tell you this as I told them. Are you ready? I need you to remember this, Stewart.

STEWART: (Nods)

THERAPIST: (places a hand on his knee, looking directly into his eyes) You did not do ANYTHING to make your Mom leave. Every kid wonders about this, but this is the TRUTH. Kids cannot do anything to make their parents go. It is not your fault. If I made the biggest mistake as a kid, it would *never* be my fault if my Mom decided to leave. I also talked to both your Mom and your Dad. I am absolutely sure she did not go away because of anything that you did. They told me that you are loved and everything they ever wanted in a son.

STEWART: (Leans heavily on the therapist, Stewart's eyes welling with tears begins to sob. After a long while, he finally speaks) Well, I couldn't think of what it was that was so bad that I did. I have been thinking so, so hard that it gave me a headache! It felt like my head was going to explode like a grenade. (makes explosive noise and softly giggles) Okay, can we play trucks now? (moving off of the couch.)

THERAPIST: Yep. Let's do it!

This session marked the moment when Stewart and I started to move into the peace cycle. He was now ready to hear the Truth. I had already identified his pain and was able to ascertain his emotionally regulating truth words. "You are loved and everything they ever wanted." He needed to know he was loved, wanted, and good enough. When these words were spoken to him, he was able to release a well of pent-up fear and emotion which brought him great relief.

He came back the next week saying he didn't feel the need to say he was sorry so much anymore. I asked him why. As he maneuvered the Tonka truck across the carpet, he replied, "because you told me it wasn't my fault, and I believed you."

I was encouraged to hear this but initially took it with a grain of salt. I continued to explore his self-shaming tendencies. I lightly peppered conversations with questions checking in to see if he was blaming himself for the abandonment. Each time I questioned him, he reassured me that he was no longer thinking this way.

Once we can build a solid rapport with a child and gain their trust, we earn the right to speak truth into their lives, and they have a remarkable sort of unwavering faith in that truth that propels them forward in their path of healing. My initial concern regarding the professionalism of finding Stewart absolutely adorable has since been answered. RT is an experiential therapy. Stewart needed to experience feeling loved, wanted, and good enough.

I genuinely welcomed, loved, and knew beyond a shadow of a doubt that Stewart was good enough. He was worthy of all of the help I could give him. If we do not have a genuine love for children who come into our office, we cannot provide a safe place for them. Kids need, more than anything else, to feel loved and secure. These are the two pillars of emotional health. If they aren't experiencing this at home, our office can be that space for them. I hope we can find something in every child that grabs our hearts and squeezes out the buckets of love due to them. If we can provide them the fertile soil of love and safety, we can stand back as they begin to grow into stable oak trees.

Stewart was my first pediatric teacher in the use of Restoration Therapy. I stood in awe as he flourished, moving from pain to peace.

Practice

After hearing Stewart's story, Let's practice the first two elements in the first objective of restoration therapy again. Please attempt to fill in the blanks here with your best guess of how Stewart feels and copes before turning the page.

Stewart Feels:

1.
2.
3.

Stewart Copes:

1.
2.
3.

Answers

Stewart Feels:

1. Unloved
2. Not good enough
3. Unwanted

Stewart Copes:

1. Shames self
2. Perfectionistic
3. Sad/depressed

Great job attempting to figure out Stewart's pain cycle was stemming from feelings of shame. Next, we will look into the flight response of escape.

Elise Escapes

Elise was nine years old, slight in frame. Her Dad was a physician, and her Mom a clergy member. Elise had wavy blonde hair and was dressed in a school uniform, checked skirt, starched white shirt, and white stockings up to her knees. Weekly, she trudged into my office in the same manner. Her head-down with a backpack that looked three times too big for her. She sluffed her backpack off of her shoulders and gave me a slight smile that left as quickly as it appeared. What's your number? I asked her. She walked to the whiteboard hanging on my office wall, picked a pink marker, and wrote a "3" on the board. She returned to sit down on the couch, and I noticed tears in her eyes. She was answering the scaling question that we used as a weekly check-in. On a scale of 1 to 10, what is your overall mood? The number 1 being horrific, "I am in the darkest saddest hole," and ten being fantastic, "I am happy and feel like I'm on top of the world!"

Elise's parents had sent her to see me because she was "sad all of the time." We had talked over some losses in her life, her grandmother, her favorite dog. We spoke of complicated friendships at school. I had met both of her parents. They were financially well off; they appeared to be in love and communicated well together in session; they were both on board with helping their daughter find her way through a peculiar sort of sadness. They briefly mentioned that Dad had dealt with feelings of depression on and off and wondered aloud if Elise was genetically predisposed. They also were very against medication and hoping it could be avoided. I observed Elise sitting very close to her Dad in session and leaning on him. He was appropriately affectionate toward her.

Elise and I drew, talked, and played together. She often appeared tired, shut down, and had a somewhat flat affect. She said she would start crying almost every other day at school and could not explain it to her teachers or friends. She described going to dinner with her family, everyone enjoying each other, but she would suddenly burst into tears. She expressed sadness, followed by a numb state. We explored further, and she said a heavy feeling would usually come over her, and she would feel like she couldn't breathe. She would then get very sad and feel as if her family would be better off without her. She said she felt like no one knew her anyway, and it would probably be easier for them if she didn't exist.

After exploring many dead-ends, I began to wonder if this would be one of my first cases, dealing with children, where the depression was organic. We had been meeting weekly for about six months, and we still weren't finding answers. The cause was frustratingly obscure. I administered a depression assessment for children. Her score indicated she was severely depressed.

I determined to tell her Mom that I thought it vitally important at this point to refer her to a psychiatrist for an evaluation. I could feel both Elise and my frustration as we were not coming up with the answers we had been searching for. As a Restoration Therapist, I looked for relational breaches in love and trust but was having difficulty pinpointing where they lay. As Elise enjoyed drawing, I decided to put a big piece of paper on my coffee table and create a genogram together. I remembered reading about the helpfulness of Genograms when needing to find answers. "Most people avoid confronting family issues because they can't see a way to change the relationships they find so frustrating." Unfortunately, it is not possible to destroy our history (McGoldrick, 1998).

We were knee-deep in re-creating her family lineage and behaviors when we uncovered a family secret that had been locked away for some time. A secret that would provide the answers we needed in discovering the source of her love or safety violation. This would start her walking on a path that would lead to healing.

THERAPIST: So, let's draw your grandmother up here on your Dad's side. What do you know about her?

ELISE: Oh, she was super nice and funny, but I don't know her well because my brother and I couldn't stay at her house for some reason.

THERAPIST: Hmmm . . . I wonder what the reason might have been? (pauses to allow time for the child to think.

ELISE: I'm not sure . . . maybe it is because my aunt is so crazy and she lived with her. She still does.

THERAPIST: Is your Dad's sister about the same age as him?

ELISE: She is two years younger, just like I am two years younger than my sister. She acts waaaaaaay younger, though.

THERAPIST: How does she act younger?

ELISE: She acts like a little kid, well not all of the time but a lot of the time, like when she was at our house for Easter, she was good during dinner, but afterward, she was singing super loud and standing on the couch.

THERAPIST: Did you sing with her? Is she fun like your grandma?

ELISE: No, she is kind of weird actually, and then I think she got sick from the ham or something because she threw up on my Dad's armchair. It was disgusting! It is my Dad's favorite chair.

THERAPIST: Oh, wow, what did your Dad do?

ELISE: Well, he was acting weird too. When his family and friends come over, they all act like dumb little kids. He was laughing, and then they all turned the music up, and he was so annoying. (her eyes filled up with tears.)

THERAPIST: (in a soft voice) I notice you are crying a little bit. What are you thinking about?

ELISE: Well, it is just makes me mad because we were having fun at lunch, and then they all started drinking different drinks, and they started acting dumb and like dumb little kids, worse than I *ever* act. My aunt asked our neighbor man who was over to kiss her, and he is married. (turning red) It was so embarrassing. My neighbor didn't kiss her though he said no and walked away, and then his wife yelled at my aunt. Oh gosh, it was terrible.

THERAPIST: Oh, my goodness. Yes, I can see how that would feel embarrassing. What did you do?

ELISE: My Mom got mad and told my brother and me to go to our room and pack some clothes. We went to my grandma's house in Montana together for almost two weeks. It was kind of fun, there was good food and I love my grandma, but I just felt that bad feeling, even more, when we were there.

THERAPIST: Does Dad drink the drinks that make him act weird a lot?

ELISE: (Long pause) Yes. I think he is that one word, maybe an Alcoholkick? I saw it on a tv show once that my Mom was watching, and she told me some people have that disease. (looks down, mumbling) I don't want him to have that disease, but he might. I didn't ask her if he does.

THERAPIST: Hmmm, I wonder how come we didn't want to ask?

ELISE: It makes me scared to talk about it. I don't want him to have a disease, but I think he does. He acts so crazy sometimes. My Mom drinks special sodas too, and my grandma, but they don't act that way. I don't know why he doesn't just stop drinking it?

THERAPIST: Yes, I wonder too. That is an excellent question. (Pointing back to the genogram) So it sounds like your aunt acts weird when she drinks, and your Dad., does anybody else?

ELISE: (nodding her head vigorously) Yes!

THERAPIST: Okay, let's take the blue marker and put a dot next to the people you have seen act weird when they drink.

ELISE: (proceeds to put a blue dot next to paternal grandpa, Dad., his brother, sister, and three of the four of her older cousins on her paternal side) It's kind of a lot of them. Oh yeah, and my Mom's Dad too. (Putting a blue dot by her maternal grandpa.) He acts like my Dad when he drinks that stuff. My Mom says he acts like her Dad and sometimes cries when she talks about it.

THERAPIST: Oh, okay. So, I wonder if your Mom might understand a little bit about how you feel? Does she talk to you about it?

ELISE: (eyes wide and answering in a whisper) No way! Nobody ever talks about it. They act like it didn't even happen. Like we came home after staying in Montana, and my parent's bed that my Dad threw up all over was clean. I don't sit on it anymore, though, but my parents still sleep there! It is disgusting.

THERAPIST: When does your Dad usually drink?

ELISE: On the weekends. He doesn't do it during the week, and I think it's because he has to go to work.

THERAPIST: Is it usually every weekend?

ELISE: Yes, and it is a lot. Like a huuuuge pack of beers in a box, and he drinks it all! I couldn't even drink that much water! Also, it was disgusting because I thought it was soda once and took a drink, and I almost gagged. That is why they throw up after they drink it. I don't know why they don't stop. (she grimaced while tears emerged)

THERAPIST: What else do you not like about it?

ELISE: It makes people act dumb, and I can't talk to my Dad. Well, I can say words to him, but he doesn't listen right or make sense, and sometimes he says things that hurt my feelings, then I get worried to be around him.

THERAPIST: Like what?

ELISE: Like last year, he said he wished I had brown eyes like my Mom's and not blue like his. He said brown eyes are prettier. He would neeevver say that if he didn't drink. I don't know if that is the truth what he said or not. So now I don't know if when he says I am pretty if he is lying or not.

THERAPIST: Yes, I imagine it seems confusing. I would stick to believing what he says when he isn't drinking. It makes us sad when people say things that hurt our feelings. I wonder if you feel sad when he is drinking?

ELISE: I feel really, really sad every single time. I don't even know why, but I do.

THERAPIST: Okay, let's try to figure it out. Let's get out some puppets. Why don't you pick the animal that you feel most like when Dad is drinking.

ELISE: Quickly picks Eddie the Escape Goat.

THERAPIST: Now, let's pick out one that reminds us of Dad when he is drinking.

ELISE: Laughs, I can't because I feel like he is the same one.

THERAPIST: Okay, no problem! I have another Eddie. (finds it for her) How about we call the one you have Edna the Escape Goat, and this will be Eddie?

ELISE: (giggles) I like Edna, she is soft and cute, and I think she is smart.

THERAPIST: (picking up Shalom the Dove and speaking through her) Can you show me what happens when you try to talk to your Dad when he is drinking?

ELISE: (speaking through Edna) Hi Dad! Can we go ice skating this weekend? (moves Eddie behind a large pillow on the couch.) Dad?? Daaaaaaaad??? Why won't you answer me? Can we please go ice-skating? (causes Eddie to peek his head out from behind the pillow) "No daughter, we can't. I am too tired, and I can't drive us there. Your eyes are ugly too." (Eddie disappears back behind the pillow)

THERAPIST: (speaking through the Dove) "Daughter goat, I can see you are so very sad. I think your eyes are beautiful. It must be hard to have your Dad drink that stuff and hide behind a pillow where you can't see him."

ELISE: (speaking through Edna in a tearful voice) "It is hard because usually my Dad is nice to me and would take me skating! I don't know if he likes me or pretends to like me when he isn't drinking."

THERAPIST: (through Shalom the Dove) That would make me feel so confused and sad too. We want our Dads to like us. Where does it hurt in your body when your Goat Dad starts to drink? What is Goat Dad saying to you when he is drinking?

ELISE: (through Edna) It hurts in my chest and my head. It feels like a thick black blanket got dropped on me. It makes me want to hide in a big dark hole and not talk to anyone.

THERAPIST: What is Goat Dad saying to you when he picks up the drink?

ELISE: (through Eddie in a slurred voice) I would rather drink this than take you skating. I love this disgusting drink the most, and you not as much! This stuff makes me throw up, and it tastes like pee and makes me mean and rude, but I don't care how you feel! (picks up Edna and begins to speak) Well, that is not nice! I hate that pee drink, and I am going to pour it on the ground outside!

(picking up Eddie and speaking) No, you are not!! (picking up Edna) Yes, I am too! You tell me nice things, and I feel safe and happy when you act normal!

THERAPIST: (speaking through Shalom the Dove) I agree with you, Edna, Daughter Goat. It hurts our feelings when people that we love choose to drink something that tastes like pee and makes them throw up. It can be *super* confusing and hard to understand. We want them to choose us and to be kind and dependable. Goat Dad., I don't think you know how your daughter, Edna, is feeling.

ELISE: (through Edna) yes, maybe you don't know how I feel, Dad.

THERAPIST: (through Shalom the Dove talking to Eddie) She said she is feeling so sad like a heavy blanket fell on her because she is confused and wondering if you will be nice or mean to her. She is right that many people she knows are almost always kind and protective of her and her feelings. Her Mom feels safe, her sister, her grandma, her friends. She is protected and cared for by all of these people. I think, Goat Dad., that you want to protect her too.

Can you look at her? She is so sad. Can you see her?

ELISE: (through Edna in a loud pleading voice) Dad!!! Can you see me? Please look at me!! I miss you when you go behind the pillow!!! Please come out and don't do that anymore!!! (Very long pause) Can we pretend that he hasn't been drinking any of that stuff now?

THERAPIST: I think that will be a wonderful thing to pretend next time. For today, we are out of time. Let's pick up our toys, and I will write it down on my paper what we will pretend he isn't drinking next time during our puppet show.

Occasionally sessions need to end abruptly. It is important to realize that this can be therapeutically appropriate. Dr. Hargrave talks about what to do if a client is in the middle of their work and we need to wrap up the session. His advice is to "immediately land the plane." At first this felt uncomfortable, frankly it still can, however, I have found time and again that this method works well, even with kids. It is helpful to process together until the last minute and wrap it up quickly. If something comes up that we think is important to revisit, it is good to note it and explore picking right back up where we left off last time. Kids respond well to this and even look forward to it. I have found it creates a strong desire to return to the next session.

Practice

From what we have observed so far in working with Elise, what might you guess is her pain cycle?

Elise Feels

   1.

   2.

   3.

Elise Copes

   1.

   2.

   3.

Answers

Elise Feels

1. Unsafe
2. Unknown
3. Unsure

Elise Copes

1. Withdraw to avoid
2. Depressed/numb
3. Critical

Great work figuring out Elise's pain cycle.

Summary

When emotional pain is ignited, some children respond with the flight response and quickly disappear into shame or escape. Although the therapist may more easily empathize with these responses, the behaviors are as destructive as the fight response. It may prove more challenging to get down to the center of their pain as the flight response creates excellent avoiders and the ability to shut down quickly. The therapist needs to hang in there and be patient using various tools, like a genogram or creative games and discussions, to uncover their core emotions that are hurting. We can see how both children in this chapter coped with their pain through the flight response. Stewart shamed himself, and Elise predominately tried to escape her pain. The coping character puppets are invaluable tools to help children externalize their problems and watch similar scenarios play out. It is important to remember that when kids display shaming tendencies, they are likely to feel unloved. Whereas, when we see escaping trends, the child is feeling unsafe. After identifying the child's pain and coping it is time to lead them into the third step of RT, the peace cycle.

References

Hargrave, T. D. (2019). *Advances and techniques in restoration therapy*. Routledge and Taylor & Francis Group.

McGoldrick, M. (1998). *You can go home again: Reconnecting with your family*. Place of publication not identified: Replica Books.

4 Identifying Love vs. Trust Violations in Children

As the world fears and mourns a global pandemic and civil unrest boils in a cauldron of confusion, seemingly ready to unleash God only knows what into our midst, it is essential to remember children's suffering. The powerless feelings that adults have are intensified for children. They are emotionally targeted by the rapid changes taking place; what they have counted on to be static and stable has become tilted and shaky. Their work areas (school) and their places of reprieve (peer interaction, playdates, theme-parks) have been shut-down.

Restoration Therapy holds to the idea that for children to move from pain to peace, they need to experience a sense of safety and love. The therapist's work helps them understand that although the world is not entirely safe, there is truth in the following ideas. 1.) The child is empowered to do something in his or her situation, 2.) The child is not alone in the type of violation he or she has experienced, 3.) The pain the child experiences through a lack of safety and tragedy will yield the fruits of strength and empowerment. These are some truths about safety where kids can cling (Hargrave, 2019).

While at a family dinner party this month, I interacted with a four-year-old extended family member; she was busy watching roller-coaster rides at Disneyland on YouTube during our chat. Her Mom shared how much her daughter loves Disneyland and has been genuinely heart-broken at the closure. In fact, for her recent birthday, her Mom lovingly set up a phone call with Mickey Mouse thinking it would bring her little one great joy. When the call went through, the family listened to the conversation. It was recounted as follows:

DAUGHTER: (smiling but with a look of concern) Mickey Mouse, can you please open up the gates of Disneyland so that I can come there?
MICKEY MOUSE: (in a Mickey Mouse voice) Well, I wish I could, but I cannot. An evil witch has cast a spell on the whole world that has made everyone sick. We can't open up our gates until we figure out a way to break the spell.
DAUGHTER: (wide eyes) okay.

DOI: 10.4324/9781003025504-4

Her Mom said it appeared to upset her more than it did her child. She could tell her daughter's wheels were turning; she didn't cry and seemed more resigned than anything. The therapist in me wanted to give Mickey Mouse's ear a yank at the observably fear inciting explanation he gave for the closure. However, the metaphor is probably more of an accurate depiction than most would like to think. The pandemic induces fear because, at least for now, it remains unpredictable, unjust, and unknown. Research shows that a sense of safety is built on opposing qualities. To feel safe, people need to experience predictability, justice or balance, and openness. Relationally, this is what is required to bring about a peaceful feeling of safety.

To help a child move from pain to peace, it is imperative to have a solid understanding of what delineates both love and trust violations, their defining factors, and the effects. When children are well-loved, they can easily rest in the reality that they are essential and significant. They can hold tight to the belief that they are wonderfully unique and valuable. When this truth that even the U.S. constitution explains is self-evident is violated somehow, an attachment injury ensues. The injurious attachment results in the form of destructive reactivity. A child is born with two fundamental basic questions: Am I loved? Am I safe? Emotional health and fortitude results if the answer is affirmative to these questions. Unsafe and unloved are the two core emotions that all other emotions spring from. When a child receives help to discover a greater sense of safety and love, first-order change will occur; these emotions of feeling unloved or unsafe lie at the epicenter of all woundedness (Hargrave & Pfitzer, 2011). One or both of these emotions are assuredly injured when a child stands before a counselor in the lobby. This is an imperative reality for any therapist to understand. The RT model explains how love and trustworthiness can be bolstered for a child. This leads to healing and relief from emotional pain. It is a fantastic discovery for anyone in the helping field.

Restoration Therapy as a Model

Restoration Therapy (RT) has been acknowledged as "The New Contextual Therapy" Terry D. Hargrave founded this theory from his studies and understanding of Boszormey Nagy's work in the field. Contextual therapy recognizes a delicate balance of giving and taking in healthy relationships, responsibility toward others, and merit for what we have offered. There is an invisible (but very real) ledger and accounting process in relational ethics (Boszormeny Nagy & Ulrich, 1981). When we give and take in relatively equal measure, trust is established. When there is a disruption in this balanced system, trust is destroyed, and feelings of guilt and or a breach in love or trustworthiness ensue (Hargrave, 2015).

From these foundational principles of Contextual Therapy, RT built a solid framework for identifying pain stemming from a lack of love or trust. When pain is present emotional dysregulation often follows unless we are

Example:

MERIT	OBLIGATION
(individual is entitled to)	(individual is expected to)

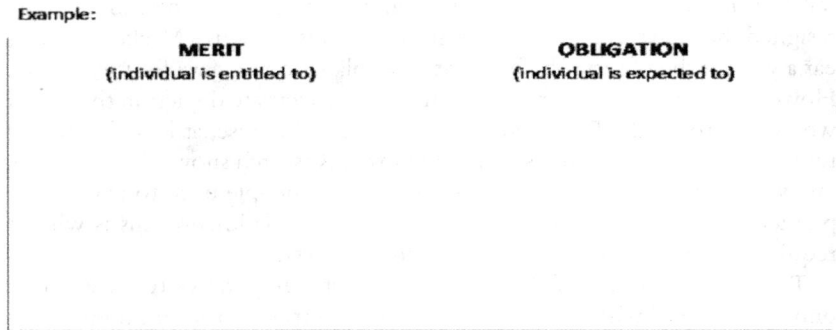

Figure 4.1 Merit Obligation chart

Figure 4.1 illustrates an example of obligation and merit typical of a working and enjoyable relationship. When one side gives and nothing is returned, a sense of anger and entitlement will likely occur. When the other side is predominately taking, the logical result is a feeling of guilt.

mindful of what is occurring and know how to effectively calm the fight or flight response (Hargrave, 2015).

A hallmark sentence that children across the globe can be heard saying (or often screaming) is "That's not fair!!" Buber (1958) first articulated that there is a relational expectation from birth that "the other" is there to provide for our relational needs. As growth occurs, we are then expected to give back. Buber discussed this philosophy in the *I and Thou relationship*. Essentially in a healthy and thriving relationship, the connection should be beneficial to both parties. RT understands that it is right and fair to expect that there be a balance of give and take.

As an RT therapist, it is good to let patients know that this equanimity is a healthy practice. There ought to be balance. It is essential to understand that people can easily trend to the extremes of being either codependent or caught in a victim or entitled mindset. Counselor and speaker, Leslie Vernick, explains that a codependent person takes on too much responsibility, feeling they can never be enough. In contrast, the person caught in a victim mindset does not take on enough responsibility. Therefore, the victim mindset leads to feeling helpless and insatiable, as if they can never get enough from the other. Not surprisingly, these two extremes tend to attract each other. This results in a painful relational dynamic followed by feelings of anger and entitlement on opposing sides. In modern-day society, entitlement invariably carries a negative connotation. However, it is a logical result of relational inequality if needs continue to be unmet. On the other hand, entitlement can become both destructive and misdirected.

Parents and Child: A Distinct Relational Ledger

Restoration Therapy mainly works from "the here and now" and moves forward experientially, but first, it is necessary to find the origin of the pain. When the child can learn more precisely the source of their suffering, they can understand they are often placing blame on the wrong person. Dr. Hargrave says destructive entitlement is often acted out in ways that make sense according to the painful feelings they experience. However, people can get caught in the act of "working with the right script and wrong players" (2015). This frequently occurs with children who have been in foster care or adopted. The child was legitimately owed love, nurture, provision, respect from their biological parent. When this responsibility was abdicated, the child will likely incur a sense of destructive entitlement even for the best reasons. This causes excellent temptation to invoke their anger and frustration onto their adoptive or foster parents. It is important to note children do not consciously do this; rather, it stems from an attachment injury. It is critical to understand that relational ethics and fairness vary drastically from spousal or peer relationships vs. the parent–child relationship.

In taking a look at relational ethics within the family system, there is an essential distinction between children and parents. The above ledger depicted a spousal or peer relationship. Likewise, when children are in relationships with peers, merit and obligation are still advisable for building healthy friendships. A youthful peer relationship may look like something like the table below:

Obligation to Give	Entitlement to Receive
1. Love	1. Love
2. Respect	2. Respect
3. Kindness	3. Kindness
4. Listening	4. To be listened to
5. Contributing toys or a favorite snack	5. Contribution of toys or favorite snack
6. Helping pick up their toys	6. Help in picking up toys

Figure 4.2 Youthful Peer Relationship Chart

This can be an excellent exercise to do with a child when explaining how to be a good friend while looking for trustworthy people to become friends with. The chart can quickly be drawn on a whiteboard or paper while allowing the child to write things within the ledger that are important to them. Again, the above two examples are how healthy horizontal or symmetrical relationships appear. There is a balanced appropriation of give and take. Giving is on one side of the ledger and receiving on the other.

However, an essential and qualitative difference occurs in vertical or asymmetrical relationships between a parent and a child.

From birth, children are vulnerable and demanding. They can't give equitably. Many parents are shocked to find their cuddly cute bundles often turn into something entirely different at three in the morning. They transform into an insatiable open mouth (and heart) that are both screaming to be fed. It is suitable for a responsible, loving parent to provide everything their child needs. This is more than a kind gesture for parents; it is an obligation. Parents tirelessly work to provide for the needs of their children. Therefore, what is the parent *owed* in return for all back-breaking, brow furrowing, sweat-filled work? The simple answer to this dilemma is nothing. The child owes the parent nothing. Of course, most parents will argue that they are blessed in many ways by their posterity; they receive connection, love, joy, eventually respect, and thanks for their efforts. The distinct difference, however, is that the parent is not rightfully owed these things. Any effort a parent puts into raising their child is rightfully for the child's benefit currently or eventually. This is why it is ineffective to punish children, yet the parent is obligated to provide discipline. The distinction between the two is imperative. Discipline is for the child's benefit, whereas punishment benefits the parent. Parents need to be mindful of this difference in motivation and be wary of demanding respect and obedience to inflate their egos or establish their own rights. Parental love and trustworthiness need to be given without condition. Only then will the child truly experience their realities. A healthy ledger balance between parent and child looks like this:

Obligation to Give	Entitlement to Receive
1. Love	1. Nothing
2. Nurture	
3. Kindness	
4. Time	
5. Provision	
6. Respect	

Figure 4.3 Healthy Parent Child Ledger

As parents pour into their children in this asymmetrical relationship, their children become full of all of the above attributes given to them. The resulting beauty is that generational justice and fairness occur. What was bestowed on the child can, in turn, be bestowed upon their children and their children's children. Therefore, although horizontal equanimity is not achieved, vertical fairness is. Most parents agree that their infant does not owe them. Unfortunately, what can often occur if a parent was not given the love, nurture, provision, or respect owed them as a child, is what RT calls destructive entitlement. More often than not, when a parent is mistreating their children and acting in an unloving or untrustworthy manner, they were deprived of their entitlements. In turn, they may feel justified in robbing their children of their birthright as well. This is a heartbreaking cycle that family therapists often feel powerless to help.

When given a chance to work with parents, who have suffered at their own parents' hands, there is good work to be done. The clinician can help the patient pinpoint this destructive intergenerational cycle. After this, they can continue to support the parent through their respective pain and peace cycles while employing reparenting exercises. Empty chair work is an example of a reparenting intervention. Once a parent can learn to care for and nurture their own heart, they can, in turn, care for and nurture their children.

Above All Else Care for Your Heart

It is essential to explain and give parents and children permission to care for their hearts first and foremost. King Solomon wrote a scripture in Proverbs 4:23. Many say he is the wisest mortal and king who ever lived. This scripture says, "Above all else, guard your heart for everything you do flows from it." It is like the familiar idea of putting our own oxygen mask on first to help others. In RT, taking care of one's heart looks like taking the time to tend to our pain by speaking what is true and practicing the four steps. Caring for ourselves first is the most important task we are given. This is an exciting concept to teach children as well as parents. As parents do the work of caring for their own hearts, the therapist can simultaneously work with the child, guiding them in the same manner. This will allow the child to experience healing from their attachment injuries. Just as little bodies trend toward rapid recovery after an injury, so do injured little minds and hearts.

Right Script Wrong Players

Now that a firm understanding of the appropriate balance of give and take has been established in both symmetrical and vertical relationships, it is essential to gain greater insight into what is meant by the "right script wrong players." When a child is robbed of what was owed him/her and parented poorly, he/she will begin to act in ways to try to earn love and safety from relationships other than his/her parental relationships. This will play out with peers and eventually significant others (Hargrave, 2019). The following is an example of how this can occur and the end result. As is depicted, it is typically unconscious on the parts of both parent and child. This is why early intervention can be helpful for both parents and children alike.

"Imagine there was a young boy who never felt like he could measure up to his musically talented older siblings. His mother, a concert pianist, often pressured him to practice as much as his older siblings and keep up with them. Due to his young age, he couldn't keep up. When he couldn't keep up, his mother would eschew him and take the family out to dinner or the theater without him. This young man labeled himself as untalented and therefore unwanted. In reality, he was exceptionally gifted and wanted. His mother did not intend for him to feel unwanted; she instead saw his raw talent, and her actions were meant to motivate him. The boy lived believing he had to perform to be welcomed and wanted. This was the "script" he thought was written for him, and he learned to play his role well. He began to work tirelessly as his need for connection was more significant than his need for rest.

He grew into a young man and fell in love with a woman who possessed a warm, easy-going kind of personality. She couldn't figure out why her husband could never seem to relax and just sit with her to watch a movie or enjoy a day off at the beach. If she walked into the living room on the rare occasion where he had dozed off to sleep, he sprung to his feet, letting her know there was a list to accomplish, and out the door, he went! This behavior became increasingly frustrating for his young wife, and no matter how often she implored him to take a break, he just couldn't seem to do it. Sensing her frustration and disappointment, he worked more tirelessly to perform. He strongly sensed this would please her, and they would be closer.

Here is an example of the right script wrong player. This young man's story and experience as a child were quite accurate. He did receive accolades, and a closer relationship was offered when he performed. His wife, however, didn't care about his performance. She cared about spending meaningful time together. Her husband was projecting his childhood experience with his mother onto the wrong player, his wife. He began to blame her for not appreciating his effort and felt that he could never be enough for her. She, in turn, felt unloved as he seemed to be ignoring her or abruptly leaving when she came into the room to spend time with him. This is an unintentional but hurtful scenario. Stories like this occur in many spousal or partner relationships. These stories stem from childhood. Had a therapist been able to work with this young man as a child, some great work could have been accomplished. His pain could have been quickly addressed at the root, saving his future relationships from many problems.

Love, Trustworthiness, and Our Family of Origin

As clinicians, we understand that the people who come to see us have experienced imperfect love and have inevitably been let down when they have trusted. If this occurs infrequently, we tend to bounce back fairly quickly and can feel generally loved. We also feel generally safe in our environment and assume it is reasonably trustworthy. However, if it happens frequently, we start to feel unsafe. In fact, what research shows us is that if love or trust is unavailable or broken even ten to fifteen percent of the time. Significant issues will arise. Terry D. Hargrave gave a poignant example of how and why this plays out. Imagine if we were looking to have a construction contractor add a bathroom to our house. If we looked at reviews on this contractor, which revealed that he acts professionally and finishes his contractual agreement 70 to 75% of the time, we would be foolish to hire him. We would assume him to be quite unreliable (2019).

Even at an eighty-five to ninety percent success rate, we would feel on edge. When parents treat their children in unloving or untrustworthy manners, more than ten to fifteen percent of the time, there will be a significant breakdown in the relationship (Hargrave, 2019). This shouldn't be surprising. To be trusted is to be reliable. It has also been pointed out that reliability is more trustworthy than intermittent kindness. For example, a child feels more stable when their parent is reliably mean-spirited. If cruel behaviors are erratic, the child is more damaged (Hargrave, 2011). When the child knows what to expect, they can rely on their agency. They can deal with the conflict more easily because they are not caught off guard. It is also imperative to have openness and vulnerability in close relationships to have trust. A child needs to be relieved from guessing what the other person wants. To be open is, to be honest about ones' own opinions, needs, desires. An open person or parent is not manipulative, and therefore a sense of security is established. Trustworthy relationships are open, just (balanced give and take), and reliable (Hargrave, 2011).

Love and safety are the pillars of what makes up an emotionally healthy child. Due to the broken world that we live in, none escape damage to these emotionally stabilizing pillars. The amount of damage falls along a continuum. The good news, however, is that reparative work can be done, regardless of the amount. The path to healing is similar in structure. Pain is an unwelcome fellow, yet an essential part of being human.

It can be argued that nothing of value comes without pain. In his new book, *David Kessler, Finding Meaning* adds a sixth stage to the initial five stages of grief, which Elisabeth Kubler-Ross founded. She is the co-author of this new work. The meaning they speak of is born from the pain of grief. Grief at its root stems from a jarring injury to our sense of love and safety. This pain, however, propels us into an opportunity that provides personal growth and greater strength once we can heal. In hindsight, after we have leaned into the work of grief, we will see we have become stronger (2020).

We will find the cracks in the pillars of Love and Trustworthiness are mended; much like human anatomy, after the healing of a broken bone, it remains reinforced and more solid than before the break. When this fellow "Pain" visits us, it helps to connect to our relationships, finding validation and hope from others' stories and experiences. The redemptive strength that is part of my childhood pain now serves as a stabilizing force. It brings me future hope and peace as I feel more assured, I will face the future when pain visits again with greater confidence. I don't look forward to it, but I know that on the other side, fortitude waits.

I was born into a family that loves me well. I have a brother four years my senior, and my parents have been married 54 years to date. I was never starved for affection or attention. My experience was quite the opposite. I was confident that I was unique and wanted. I am thankful for this gift and don't often suffer from a low sense of self. I believe that I matter to the people who most matter to me. I think I am relatively well-liked and feel warmly welcomed into most circles. I recall my paternal grandmother looking out the window, watching for me to come to her house every time I arrived. She had a long gravel driveway, and before I was old enough to see out of the car window, I felt the rush of rocks spinning underneath tires, and my heart would pound excitedly. When the car stopped, I would scramble to my knees and spot my Grandma in the window, drapes pulled back, a broad smile on her face, as quickly as I saw her, she would disappear to rush out to meet me, showering me with words of affirmation and kisses.

What a way to be greeted as a kid! There was not a doubt in my mind that my presence was significant to my Grandma; I was cherished. I often think of her example when I greet kids in the lobby of our practice. I, of course, cannot be so demonstrative, yet I want them to feel my delight in welcoming them. My desire is for them to know that they truly matter, and I am intentional that my facial expressions and words reflect this to them. My parents, brother, grandparents, aunts, uncles, and cousins are overarchingly loving, resulting in my belief that I am lovable and worthy of being loved. This is something I am eternally grateful for. I was indeed well-loved, but I lived with a sense of feeling very unsafe.

Growing up, I believed there were only a small handful of people that I could trust and that the few I could, were predominantly women and not men. My Mom came from a traumatic environment of sexual and spiritual abuse. Her mother died when she was nine years of age. Her father was left alone to raise seven children and became detached and unavailable in his grief. This left the younger four children in the family vulnerable to horrendous abuse. In turn, the four youngest children suffered from prolonged episodes of major depression and suicidality. All of this caused a lot of anxiety in me. Abusers don't often realize the scope and length of the painful impact they cause. There is almost always a generational ripple effect, and perpetrators need to be held accountable. I do not blame my mother for her hyper-vigilant responses. She was doing her best to protect me and has since humbly apologized for the pain it caused in my life. I firmly believe she has always only wanted what was in my best interest. I share my story because it has helped me honor the pain children often carry. I have been able to look back and appreciate what my parents, grandparents, and other mentors brought into my life to help me heal as a child and beyond. However, there were hard times, and I remember the painful feelings that seemed to leave me at a loss to find peace.

I cried every day of the first grade and was given awards in class if I could dry my tears for even half of the day. I often felt incredibly unsafe and responsible for helping my Mom through her emotions. I had the genuine fear of coming home to a dead mother lying on our couch. I knew the reality of my uncle's suicide that he left his daughter and family alone because life became too sad for him. I was apprised of my aunt's many attempts. Suicide was a real part of my young life, and it became vital that I was able to cheer my Mom up. I did not always know how to do this, but I tried my best. I figured out how not to upset her and to be a reliable comforter. I could do this much. I knew that I was much safer with her than without her, and I loved her very much. I did not know what I would do or how I would be taken care of without a mother. Much of my Mom's energy was used to make my life better than hers had been, and she was successful in a considerable measure.

She knew that all of the secrets in her home as a child were unhealthy. She felt obligated to inform me so that I could be vigilant about protecting me. It was partially effective but left me with copious amounts of anxiety and fear. Although unintended, it felt as if it fell on me to carry this load with her daily. Oh, how I wished I could be enough to help, but I sorely sensed my inadequacy. A seasoned professional therapist rendered my mother's story the most tragic she had heard; imagine the burden that was placed on my six-year-old shoulders. I was told not to talk about it. This resulted in what Dr. Joy Osofsky, a renowned pediatric psychiatry professor, describes secondary trauma, often transmitted from mothers to daughters (2011). On the bright side, along with loving me well, my Mom instilled in me a strong knowledge and faith in God. As a little girl, it sometimes felt my only safe forms of expression were writing and praying to my most comforting friend, Jesus.

Often, when my Mom was severely depressed and fear weighed on me too heavily, I would retreat to an empty large white wall in our house. It stood near the stairwell. On this blank canvass, I would use my finger to write my feelings, invisibly, on the wall. I imagined my writing in various Crayola colors. I knew that Jesus and I were the only people who could see the words I wrote on that wall. It was significant to me that he read them. I can still envision many of them there. This worked to ease my pain and anxious insecurities. Because much of my Mom's abuse included people I interacted with, I was groomed not to trust people easily. This left me feeling powerless. I believed her, though, when she told me that I could trust Jesus. I saw him at work in my Mom's life; I felt his love for me. I constantly talked to him, and most importantly, I believed he could keep me safe. He was my Savior and my sanity on many suffocating nights. I often slept with my Children's Bible on the pillow beside me, recalling the verse "I will never leave you or forsake you" (Joshua 1:15, NIV). My faith is still a profound core value, and I resource it daily, finding peace and comfort.

My Mom's depression caused a sort of closeness with my brother that many little sisters lack; he was/is an extraordinary brother and often helped me bear the weight of responsibility that I felt. He did not know the entirety of our Mom's story, but he knew of her sadness and my fear. He cared for me while we both cared for our Mom the best he could. We are still close, and probably not surprisingly, we are both licensed therapists. I have to smile at the redemptive nature of painful experiences. If we allow our pain to be used, it finds itself useful every single time.

Growing up, my father was jovial and a hard worker. He gave me abundant amounts of appropriate affection whenever he was around. My Dad had a particular nomadic nature about him. We had moved 18 times by the time I was 18 years of age. Looking back, each time we had to move, my Mom had to rally. She had to pack us up, move us in and get us settled. It was something she was good at. Because of our many moves, I was always the new girl. This had both a positive and negative effect on my life. I became very good at making friends and also saying goodbye to friends. I became adept at reading people to fit into the various cultures that I was placed in. Along with my Dad., I enjoyed some of the adventures and challenges of this type of lifestyle, but I also often felt painfully unknown.

My husband, Rick, describes his childhood experience as quite the opposite of mine. He felt incredibly safe with nary a worry in the world. He only moved once during his first 19 years of life, and then just a block away from their previous house, of which they maintained ownership. His Dad was a Doctor of Chiropractic who owned the same practice for 40 years. His parents were well-to-do, and he never imagined being concerned with money or stability. His Dad was so predictable in word and deed that others around him wished he were more spontaneous and emotionally reactive. For instance, he set reminders on his calendar to prompt him of the exact time to write his Mom a love-note or to buy her flowers.

Rick struggled with feeling significant and loved as a child. Although he felt safe, he worried about being wanted, especially by his father. His Dad did certain things extraordinarily well. He was a generous provider and worked tirelessly for the physical needs of his family. Like all of us, he did, however, miss the mark in certain areas. My husband has a starkly different personality than his Dad., and his Dad seemed to lack the ability to bond with him or make him feel like he could measure up. We have since learned of my husband's ADHD and suspect that my father-in-law was somewhere on the autism spectrum. Like oil and water, my father-in-law displayed high predictability, low emotionality with some apparent sensory issues. On the other hand, my husband was born an extreme extrovert who was very entertaining, loud, impulsive, spontaneous, and fairly emotional. It was trying to create an emotional connection between the two.

Rick's Mom was naturally a nurturing, loving woman. However, she had four children in four years; my husband is the youngest. He has identical twin sisters almost two years older, and his brother is three and a half years older. His mother's job of trying to make up for his Dad's lack of nurture and emotion must have felt insurmountable. These are wonderful people that I speak of; however, my point is that when Rick and I met, we each suffered profoundly from our attachment wounds from childhood.

Furthermore, the wounds we suffered were extremely opposite, much like our personalities. I felt remarkably loved. My husband felt exceptionally safe. These are beautiful blessings; however, we did not easily recognize the woundedness of the other. This created great misunderstandings resulting in pain and confusion. This nebulous pain would propel us into a crazy cycle of hurting each other despite overarchingly good intentions. We were responding out of our childhood pain and patterns of coping. We had been steeped in these behaviors for years before we even met. It was an "aha" moment for both of us when we realized the pain we suffered did not originate within our marriage but rather our childhoods. We had been acting in the right script but substituting the wrong players. Thankfully, Rick and I attended RelateStrong, a training that Sharon Hargrave facilitates. This training helped us apply the four objectives of RT to our marriage and see how the Pain and Peace Cycle's work against and for our relationship. We found it extraordinarily helpful.

I only wish we had a therapist who understood these developing patterns at five and six years old. Our stories fuel the passion for helping little ones learn healthier approaches. It is interesting because observing and trying to treat my childhood issues from the typical family therapy model of the top-down approach would have proven problematic. I honestly do not believe my Mom was able to do personal work when I was that young. I think she was still too close to the hot coals of her pain to see straight. As a very young Mom, she was still entrenched in her trauma. If someone could have seen me, though, a therapist who knew what questions to ask and how to guide me, I have no doubt it would have been life-changing, and the help seared in my memory. I had moments of times like this when I was young. Times when other people spoke into my life, and I can attest to their impact.

"Trusted Adults Can Have a Lasting Impact on a Child's Emotional Health."

Trusted adults can have a lasting impact on a child's emotional health. I believe I likely would have suffered from OCD as a teenager and maybe an adult if it weren't for my grandmother. I recall being on a trip to visit her. I had great difficulty being away from my mother as I feared for her very life. I loved my grandmother so dearly, though, that I put up with the anxiety to visit. I remember having a lot of trouble going to bed and falling asleep without overwhelming fears. I had taken to performing an unhealthy ritual of brushing my teeth in a specific pattern. I then would rinse my mouth ten times, followed by cupping my hand and drinking precisely five drinks from the faucet. At the age of ten, I remember thinking that someone in my family would die if I did not follow through with this ritual. It would likely be my Mom or me. I experienced that this ritual was giving me some sort of strange relief.

When my Grandma questioned why I was in the bathroom for so long, I trusted her enough to tell her. "Well, I have to brush my teeth and then rinse ten times, then I drink five gulps of water from my hand. If I don't do it, I feel like my Mom or me, or maybe even you might die. So, I have to do it." "Oh, Nancy," she said, wrapping me in her arms and frowning. "That just isn't the truth, and I don't want you to do that anymore because some people get stuck doing those things, and they can't stop. Can you promise me you will stop doing that? We can brush our teeth together differently tomorrow, and no one is going to die. I promise." "What are you so afraid for, Sweetie?" I couldn't articulate it and answered, "I don't know." I cried, and she hugged me tighter. "Do you want me to sleep next to you tonight? Grandpa won't care." "Yes," I said. "Can you tell me stories about when you were a little girl?" "Yes, I will. Do you want a lemon drop even though you just brushed your teeth?" She giggled, and I nodded yes.

I clearly remember lying next to her, a little afraid that I couldn't follow the new routine that brought me relief the next day. Something in me believed her that my ritual would not make a difference regarding who lived or died. I even knew she was there to walk beside me as I tried something different. True to her word, she appeared beside me in the bathroom the next night with her toothbrush. If she could be faithful to her word, then so could I. I think this was a pivotal moment and a crisis point in my mental health. Although, I continued, and truthfully still do struggle with anxiety. I did not return to OCD tendencies. I believed my Grandma to be truer than my temptations. I was able to relinquish the desire to control my anxiety in this regard because I trusted her. The pattern was relatively easy to break. I had not practiced for long, and I had someone I loved and trusted to help walk beside me and step onto a peaceful path. My grandmother was

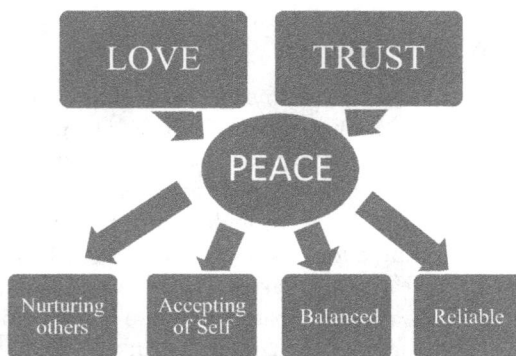

Figure 4.4 Individual Peace Cycle

far from being a therapist, but she helped my young neuro-pathways trend toward peace by being both a loving and trustworthy influence.

Figure 4.4 Individual Peace Cycle is an illustration showing how an environment of love and trust fosters peace. This is an ideal environment. It depicts the natural behavioral outcomes that flow out of a relationship filled with love and trust are nurturing others, valuing the self, balanced give and take, and reliable engagement.

When love and trust have not been established, our feelings and subsequent behaviors become maladaptive. Before we move into the following chapters and vignettes observing therapist and client interaction, it is essential to remember the four objectives that the therapist moves through during the therapeutic process. They are as follows:

1.) Define and understand the pain
2.) Identify the truth
3.) Emotionally regulate using client truths
4.) Mindful Practice—Here is where we systematically explain the theory

Objectives

We have already discussed the first objective being imperative to understand the client's woundedness source. In line with this objective, to define and understand pain, it is essential to know that conflict equals pain. The brain registers the emotional pain that results from the conflict in the same region where it registers physical pain. When pain occurs, the brain signals warnings (Hanna, 2014). The warning originates from an actual or perceived feeling of being unloved or unsafe.

During our discussions and assessments of children, we are searching to discover precise, painful feelings. Does the child feel alone, unprotected, powerless, or unloved, unworthy, inadequate? We can determine this through a variety of interventions. The most effective way is to see how the client is employing destructive coping methods and move back to their reason for their coping. For instance, if a client tends to react by blaming others or shaming the self, this can be traced back to a love violation. Meaning, this particular child likely has struggled to feel loved, important, or significant. They often wonder if they matter.

On the other hand, if the child is reacting by controlling or escaping, they likely have suffered a breach of trust. These particular children struggle to feel safe and wonder if anyone has their back. When we can help equip a child with defining words most aptly describing their pain, this validates their experience and helps them uncover the reasoning behind their troublesome coping methods. We can validate that it makes sense they are trying to distract or soothe these painful emotions. However, coping in destructive ways only further the pain cycle. Understanding the child's pain and its origination is key to helping effectively. The coping is inevitably more straightforward to identify than the pain. The four types of coping are as follows:

Blame

Certain children react with a blame or anger response. Rick's childhood story and attachment injury ignited feelings within him of being unloved or unimportant. These feelings caused him to respond to relational conflict by accusing others, not taking responsibility, or saying it was someone else's fault. This pattern of his brought into our marriage from childhood proved to frustrate and bewilder me to no end! Had I known these behaviors stemmed from a wounded identity, I could have been a more understanding partner.

Shame

The second response from this type of emotional pain in conflict is a shame response. The shame responder typically feels as if everything is his/her fault. If they had done something differently, the fight would not have happened. People who go to shame often feel bad about themselves and who they are as a person.

Control

The third response that was discussed was the controlling response. When in pain, some people will start telling other people what they need to do, that they are the only ones with the correct answers, and others should think as they do. The more introverted personality does not always seek to control others but will seek to control their environment by perfectionistic or performing tendencies. They can have an over-inflated sense of self-control. The controlling response can manifest in codependent caretaking. This is a tendency for people in helping professions and for many therapists.

Escape

The fourth and last response is the escape response. An "escape response" is typically displayed by looking for various ways to escape during a conflict. My childhood attachment injury resulted in me feeling unsafe. Escape has been my go-to destructive coping mechanism. For me, this can look a lot like shutting down, zoning out, leaving the room, getting in my car and driving away, or perhaps losing myself in work. For some, escape takes on addictive forms such as alcoholism, excessive shopping, exercise, drugs, or pornography.

The RT model asserts that when people are hit with feeling unloved, unsafe, inadequate, powerless, alone, or rejected, they will respond in one of these four ways. They are part of the fight or flight response. They also reminded us that it was necessary to remember that these responses nearly always originated from childhood or adolescent experiences (Hargrave, 2011). This is helpful information to relay to a child; it can alleviate feelings of blame and guilt. It helps them realize they are common issues.

The Source of Pain

The painful feelings we experience come from one of three sources: our family of origin, experiences we have while growing up, or people and peers outside of our family (Hargrave, 2011). For instance, those who grew up with much tragedy within their families will likely feel unsafe, like my mother's experience. If there is physical, verbal, emotional, or sexual abuse, our sense of self-worth will be attacked, and we will likely struggle with feeling unsafe as well as unloved. However, it is interesting to note that people tend to lean more toward either a struggle to feel loved or a struggle to feel safe. Even when they have experienced extreme breaches in both love and trustworthiness from their family of origin, they typically find that one is more problematic than the other.

Furthermore, we experience situational traumas in the growing up years that can also affect us, causing wounds. Even if our family was very trustworthy and loving, we might have had to deal with extreme financial hardship, a house fire, school shooting, medical issues, or like kids today, a global pandemic and civil unrest.

The third possible reason for our pain's origin may well have been learned emotional responses from harm by someone outside of our family. For example, suppose we consistently hear negative messages about who we are. We can also feel perpetually unsafe by being bullied at school or enduring teasing for various issues. Kids can endure pain from being over or underweight or feeling like they don't measure up athletically, socially, academically, or musically.

From whichever source the pain originates, it can significantly impact our core beliefs about who we are and cause us to question our safety. When we question our identity and safety, it plays out visually like the chart below: The violation of love or trust results in pain and confusion. This pain and confusion cause feelings of either being unloved or unsafe. If we are feeling unloved, we respond by blaming others or shaming ourselves. When we feel unsafe, we react by attempting to control others or ourselves, or we go into escaping behaviors. This visual construct is a helpful reminder of the process that is occurring. At a point, it may be beneficial to show this to a parent or child. Another option is to draw a version of it together in session.

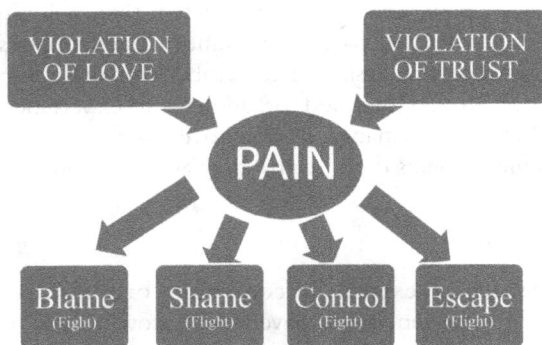

Figure 4.5 Individual Pain Cycle

Wounds and Scars

We carry these wounds throughout life. We might make it a habit to explain to children the difference between wounds and scars. We first question them about a time they have been physically hurt. It is not uncommon for kids to have an unhealed scrape or sore; they are physically active and still learning how to maneuver their growing frames safely. Over 50% of the time, they seem to have something hurting, and they are usually quite excited to launch into a "show and tell." Identifying their physical injuries works remarkably well. We ask them to describe the pain then and now. They usually use words like "burning, stinging," shocks of lightning, etc. . . . we then question what it would be like if someone were to poke it. They are typically incredulous at such a suggestion. We could follow with a question of how it would feel. Typically, the answer is that it would hurt, and they would feel angry or sad. We follow with a question of how they would react? Some may reply that they would hit the other person or tell them they should not be so mean and stop, while others may cry and run away.

This is often a first peek into their pain cycle. They are hurt, they feel, they react. We discuss scars as a foreshadowing of the peace cycle. Ask them if they have a scar that we can see. Kids invariably tend to find many of them. They will point to a scar on their knee, ankle, finger, eyebrow. We can ask them to poke their scar. They usually proudly poke their scars and tell me how it doesn't hurt anymore. We inquire how they may respond if their Mom, Dad., or sibling poked their scar. They seem to like this question as well and say things like. "I wouldn't care at all, or they can touch it all they want!"

This proves to be an experiential exercise for kids and one they can understand. We can then correlate this experience to emotional pain, and interestingly enough, they often use the same vocabulary to describe both emotional and physical pain (Hanna, 2014). This should not be surprising, knowing the brain views emotional and physical pain somewhat synonymously.

When our wounds from childhood are not yet healed, we naturally become reactive and emotionally dysregulated due to being thrust into the fight or flight response (Hargrave, 2019).

If we could only teach early on how to regulate these painful emotions by telling ourselves the truth at a younger age, we could save our clients much heartache. This is a process we can absolutely teach to children!

References

Boszormeny-Nagy, I., & Ulrich, D. N. (1981). Contextual family therapy. In A. S. Gurman & D. P. Kniskern (Eds.), *Handbook of family therapy* (pp. 159–186). Brunner/Mazel.

Buber, M. (1958). *I and thou.* Charles Scribner and Sons.

Hanna, S. M. (2014). *The transparent brain in couple and family therapy: Mindful integrations with neuroscience.* Routledge.

Hargrave, S. (2011). *Building marriages for life and leadership.* The Hideaway Foundation.

Hargrave, T. D. (2015). *New contextual therapy: Guiding the power of giving and take.* Routledge.

Hargrave, T. D. (2019). *Advances and techniques in restoration therapy.* Routledge and Taylor & Francis Group.

Hargrave, T. D., & Pfitzer, F. (2011). *Restoration therapy: Understanding and guiding healing in marriage and family therapy.* Routledge.

Kessler, D. (2020). *Finding meaning: The sixth stage of grief.* Scribner.

Osofsky, J. D. (2011). *Clinical work with traumatized young children.* Guilford Press.

5 Helping Children Regulate Emotions and The Peace Cycle

After the client's pain is accurately identified, the next step is to help the client recognize the truth about their identity and sense of safety. This chapter is full of creative ideas for play that will furnish the therapist with ways to help children challenge their painful feelings by experiencing the truth about their value and sense of safety. When kids experience peace from the reality of their safety and identity, brain activity changes, and new neurological pathways form. These truth messages allow the child to learn to get in touch with a deep sense of calm (Hanna, 2014). At this point, destructive coping is no longer needed, and the therapist encourages an experience of new alternative behavior. This new behavior reinforces the peaceful state that the child is experiencing, and a beneficial form of circular causality occurs.

Thus far, we have been invited into the therapeutic room with several pediatric patients. Hopefully, we are familiar and somewhat practiced in identifying the first two elements in the initial objectives of Restoration Therapy (identifying pain and coping). The second goal is to identify the truth which induces emotional regulation. Let's explore how to help the client move to this stage.

Just as our pain typically stems from one of three places, so do our beliefs about the truth (Hargrave, 2011). It is imperative to help the patient challenge painful beliefs and feelings. We saw an example of this when talking with Stewart; he was living under the assumption that he was unloved, could never say he was sorry quite enough, and therefore believed *he* was not enough. He was convinced he was unwanted. The truth was that his parents absolutely wanted him. Although his mother was lost in drug addiction, she continued to fight for custody and visitation.

We can help children find freedom by letting them know they choose to react destructively or constructively when painful feelings come. It is beneficial to discuss with children what they can change and what they cannot. It helps to talk about having a choice to respond to all of our feelings, no matter what! Kids can follow this logic quite well, and it is profitable to brainstorm ways that they have already accomplished this practice of making positive choices. Collaboratively processing how we can challenge our feelings is great to explore, explain, and play out with the coping puppets.

DOI: 10.4324/9781003025504-5

A Journey to Discover the Truth

Something that I have discovered works quite well for kids as we move into the second objective of Restoration Therapy is to invite kids by using toys or puppets whom they identify with, on "an exploration to find the truth about themselves." We can let them know we will journey to three places where we can find out this truth. They will visit friends (others), spiritual resources (God or a Higher Power if they have religious beliefs), and the mirror (themselves). The puppets can learn new things about themselves at each part of their journey, and they can revisit these places as often as they wish. This interactive "journey" helps kids recognize and remember the three areas where they can discover the truth.

As with Stewart, when he sought the truth from others, his therapist, his Dad., and eventually, his Mom, he was reassured that his feelings of being unloved, not good enough, and unwanted were not accurate. The truth he discovered was that he was dearly loved, good enough, and very much wanted. Stewart's Dad also took him to church, and true to form, what he found most helpful in the church were the lyrical messages in the songs. He quickly memorized them and excitedly relayed the various songs he learned. He mentioned a song where Jesus invited him to be a "fisher of men and to follow him." He excitedly explained that Jesus welcomed everyone to come along, even if they had made mistakes or had done something terrible. This idea resonated deeply with Stewart as he very much liked the idea of being welcomed and wanted. We discussed this at some length. He then excitedly let me know that there was another account of a guy named Peter in the Bible, one of Jesus's friends, who made some big mistakes, but Jesus said: "Don't worry Peter, I still love you, and you can be my friend." The truth messages that Stewart was loved and wanted were essential messages that Stewart learned from spiritual resources. If we discover a client's spirituality, children included, it can invariably be used as a resource to help shape identity and a sense of safety. "The therapist does not need to be an expert on all spirituality or religions for use as helpful resources. They only need to be curious and interested" (Hargrave & Pfitzer, 2011).

The third source for discovering the truth is the self. Using Stewart's example, we see that the self is likely an essential tool we have at our disposal. The self is what incites and sustains lasting change. Other people can speak an abundance of truth into our lives; however, if we choose not to believe them, the message will not take root. This idea applies to spiritual resources. If we lack faith and choose not to believe in what any creed or book says, the truth will not reach us. In accepting any form of truth, we must look to ourselves and decide to believe others or what our faith teaches. We also are free to determine what our mind believes about who we are. I value the saying, "we are the boss of our brain." We can choose to accept accurate messages about ourselves.

This journey of discovering the truth is far more in-depth than learning to muster positive affirmations and self-talk. It requires a firm, decisive action to explore our pain courageously. Followed by the vulnerable, often terrifying search to discover the reality about who we are at our very core. This part requires humbly accepting feedback from others, our faith, and ourselves. Finally, we must take action to change our self-talk and change our behaviors as well.

Positive affirmations and self-talk are good practices, but often people don't actually believe the words they are saying to themselves. They are the boss of their brains; however, it is difficult to outsmart the brain perpetually (Hargrave, 2019). When people intentionally take the arduous journey to discover the reality of who they are, they find their actual value. They simply need to remind their brains of what they are convinced is already the truth. This conviction brings a sustaining sense of peace.

I appreciate Pia Mellody's explanation that value is intrinsic and a static concept (Mellody, 1989). I regularly use her visual methodology with children who are questioning their value and worth in session. In adapting this exercise for use with children, it looks something like this: Draw a straight line across the middle of a whiteboard or a piece of paper. Write "value" or "worth" on the line. Explain that there is a big gigantic lie that many people tell us. The lie is that our worth or value can change depending on things that we have or do. Ask the child to help name some things that people might give us more worth or value. Kids often say something like, "being pretty, having a certain type of bicycle, getting a lot of presents, having lots of people like us, being good, being an athlete or good at drawing." The therapist can write all of these phrases above the value line. After this is finished, ask what people believe makes someone worth less? They may say things like "not having any toys, not being good at video games or baseball or soccer, getting in trouble, not helping, being a bully, taking drugs, being ugly or not having nice clothes, etc. . ." As they rattle these off, write them below the value line. Tell them that all of the things above and below the value line are just differences. Differences do not make us worth more or less than anyone else. Both adults and children become skeptical at this point. Allow time for them to think this through.

The following is a story that I use to illustrate my point. My husband Rick is a masterful storyteller. He came up with this story about intrinsic value when working in a juvenile detention center for girls. Many incarcerated girls have suffered severe abuse throughout their lifetime. This population persuasively struggles with feeling like they have worth, dignity, or value. I tell this story to adults and children, changing it slightly according to age and attention span (I typically only do this value exercise or share the following story with nine-year-olds or older). It has consistently proved a helpful intervention. The story goes as follows:

> Can I tell you a story to help us understand something about how every single person on the planet has value? Imagine with me that we are going to walk out to the lobby after we finish our session. Can you

picture it? When we get to the waiting area, we see a Dad sitting there with a four or five-month-old baby. Let's imagine this baby together and picture her. (I typically match the baby's gender to the gender of the client) Do you see her/him? This little baby girl has her socks off because it is hot here in Phoenix, and we can see her little toes wiggling. She sees them wiggle too and reaches down to grab them with her chubby hands. She looks up at us and smiles while she puts her newfound foot into her mouth.

We smile at her while she says something to us in her baby language. Her Dad., who has been paying attention to his phone, glances down at her and sighs in disgust. "Ew! You are one disgusting kid. Get your foot out of your mouth!" He impatiently unbuckles her from her car carrier and picks her up. She immediately spits up what looks like half of a bottle of milk all over his shoulder and arm. Her Dad holds her out from him and, looking into her face, glares at her. "You are the worst baby ever! What a horrible kid. How did I get stuck with you?" At his words and tone, the baby begins to cry loudly. "Shut up, you stupid kid!" We watch his anger grow while the little one's cries grow louder.

We now notice the baby has dirtied its diaper, and the contents are leaking onto her Dad's arm. When the father sees this, he begins to curse at the child, tossing it roughly back into the car seat; he slaps it hard across the face—the baby screams."

Lowering my voice, I continue. "I want you to notice your emotions. What are you feeling watching this all happen?" I allow a long pause here to enable time for the client to form their thoughts.

"Okay, now I would like you to come back to this room and talk to me. What were you feeling?" Usually, I get responses like, "I am so mad and angry!" or "I felt very sad for that little baby. It isn't the baby's fault." I usually interrupt a statement like this, saying, well, wasn't it the baby's fault that it was chewing on her feet or that it threw up? Dad didn't throw up or poop on his own arm." I usually get an exasperated look here, and the response is something like, "Well, that is just what babies do." "Isn't that disgusting, though?" I reply. "Well, I guess, yes, but still, she is just a baby, and she isn't disgusting!" "Okay, I reply, she may *do* some disgusting things, but you don't think she *is* disgusting?" "No. she is not!" they reply.

"Would you say she is valuable?" I offer. "Yes! she is super valuable." "Hmmm, how do we know she is valuable? Let's look back at our list to see if she is valuable or not. Does she have a nice bicycle, no? Does she get good grades, no? Is she good at soccer or the best at playing video games? I wonder if she does a lot of good things to help people?" I usually pause and wait for their response. It is intriguing to hear a child's response here. They typically become pretty adamant about letting me know that these things do not matter. I challenge them in a friendly manner, saying things like, "she can't do anything except throw up on people and wake people up screaming in the middle of the night. She is often stinky and not helpful but causes everyone to help her. Are you sure she is worth anything? Kids and adults alike typically get very animated, trying to convince me of the reality of the worth of this little baby.

It is impressive to hear the kids voice all of the reasons and then land on the idea that her worth is not dependent on what she does or doesn't do. Her value and worth are based on her being human. After a child arrives at this place, I agree whole-heartedly, letting them know they have discovered a treasure and the treasure is to know the truth about human value. We talk about many people believing the lie that our differences make us more or less valuable.

I inevitably end the intervention in the following manner: (speaking softly again and leaning forward in my chair) Okay, I would like us to imagine this baby one more time. Close your eyes with me, and let's picture her. She is crying from her Dad screaming at her and calling her worthless and disgusting. Her Dad has left her alone. Now you go over and, with a clean blanket, pick up that baby very gently. What do you say to the baby? The child may say something to the effect of, "Hi little baby, you are so cute, and I am sorry that your Dad yelled at you and was very mean. You are precious and important, and I will take care of you." "Wow, those are wonderful things to tell that baby."

Now, imagine with me that you are that baby. Have you seen pictures of what you looked like when you were little? "Tell me what you looked like?" Allow the child to describe themselves and repeat their description while you speak. "Okay, so I am imagining looking at this little baby that is you. It has just a little bit of dark brown hair and big brown eyes. It has chubby rosy cheeks and a cute little nose. I'd like you to tell your wonderful baby self some of those nice things again." "You are so cute . . ." pause to allow the child to complete your sentence. "you are precious, you are important, you are wonderful, and I will take care of you." If the child uses a soft tone, match their tone and say, "now imagine how this little baby is feeling hearing all of these kinds, good and true words. How does the baby feel?" "The baby feels comfortable and happy and safe." The child replies. Now we can repeat these words and pause to let them sink in. This typically proves to be a sacred experience with patients as they must call on their internal sources of compassion and own sense of intrinsic value.

The reality is that each one of us is the baby in this illustration. We are born priceless; any mother or father in their right mind would give their life for their child, as would many strangers. We can do nothing to earn or lesson our value. We can make choices that have consequences that affect our quality of life, but our worth is not dependent on what choices we make.

This experiential exercise can be adapted to use with young and old alike. It is something that all can experientially and intuitively understand. It also offers excellent insight into what their peace cycle is. We find that clients usually speak their desired truths presenting their pain messages' antithesis during this exercise. When the therapist repeats this to them after they say it to themselves, clients can hear it from others, the self, and a soulful or spiritual place. If the child does not have the attention span to engage the length of this intervention, we can efficiently act this scenario out with dolls. It is fantastic to see them rush to protect and speak the truth to themselves in this setting. This experiential form of guided imagery is a practical example of helping a child access their truth messages. Sometimes, with established rapport and trust, children, more readily than adults, will simply believe the truth when they hear it.

As we may recall in the case of Stewart, when he looked into my eyes, he made the internal choice to believe me at my word, "It is not your fault that your Mom left." His belief brought him great relief. He started to sleep better; he experienced peace because he maintained that he was loved, good enough, and wanted. He accepted these words to be accurate. After he made this internal decision, it was reinforced by others and spiritual resources from the church where he attended. Within this process, Stewart pushed through the Lying Lizard's messages and the subsequent flight response. How did he do this? He became the "boss of his brain" by challenging his feelings and believing the truth.

Challenging, painful beliefs with the truth is precisely what the six-year-old girl in the Olympic-sized pool did. She pushed through her pain by reassuring herself of what was real. She was then able to respond productively by swimming the entire length without taking a breath. She *chose* to believe the truth that her trusted father spoke into her. In so doing, she defeated the Lying Lizard and pushed through the unhelpful fight or flight response.

Ancient biblical wisdom addresses this idea of truth regulating us and, in turn, enabling us to live unhindered lives. Jesus is recorded in (John 8 vs. 32) "Then you shall know the truth, and the truth will set you free." Jesus, who is argued to be the wisest man who ever walked the earth, touted this concept. When children get to this part of the Restoration Therapy process, it is an exciting time. It is remarkable and rewarding to see how they overcome their pain and start moving into peace.

Once again, the second goal of restoration therapy is to guide our clients into discovering the truth about themselves. Regulating truth is found through others, spiritual resources, and the -self (Hargrave, 2019). Once the truth is discovered, self-regulation occurs naturally. It doesn't have to be mustered up or fought for through a white-knuckled approach. In receiving the truth, with open hands, the result is relaxed peace.

Fortunately, this isn't quite the end of the story. We still need a bit more practical application to keep us moving in a positive direction. There are two more necessary steps to walk through. We need to identify the Peace cycle and practice moving from pain to peace by employing the four steps.

Because our brain is a creature of habit, when we have habitually replayed and reenacted the pain cycle, it takes some directed work to rewire our thoughts and responses. Initially, we can expect it to prove challenging to remain in the place of peace, where truth and emotional regulation reign supreme.

The following chart can be used to help both the therapist and child identify their truth and action words:

Prince of Pain and King of Peace Activity

One way to help set up this idea of needing to move from pain to peace that resonates with children is by using army men and battle scene toys to create an enactment that will establish the need and illustrate the process. We can explain that there are two rulers in the land where we live. One ruler is named the Prince of Pain. When he is allowed to be in charge, the people fight a lot because they feel (enter the child's top three painful feeling words here) unsafe, unloved, and unwanted. When the people in the land feel this way, they do things like (enter child's specific coping methods) throw tantrums, get angry, and feel bad about themselves. The residents hate living in this land when the Prince of Pain is in control. The good news is that there also is a King of Peace. In this land, the people know that they are (enter child's truth) safe, loved, and wanted. When they know this, they don't fight with each other; instead, the people are (enter child's actions) easy going, kind and happy with who they are.

We can set up the army men with a throne center stage as we explain these different lands. We can work together to develop various strategies for capturing the Prince of Pain and locking him up. After we catch him, we can explain that as soon as the people start to fight, the Prince of Pain will escape captivity and sit back on the throne. The people will then have to remind themselves of the truth, reciting their truth words over and over. This will cause the Prince of Pain's power to weaken and free the King of Peace to sit back on the throne.

We can get very creative within this basic script. I have found that by personalizing the battle using the child's specific feeling, coping, and truth words. It is impressive what buy-in we will get. This intervention also ushers in the third step of identifying the peace cycle.

Step Three: The Peace Cycle

After the child begins to learn the truth about themselves, the next step is to move into how the new behaviors will look. Rather than acting out like Brutus the Blaming Badger, Sharla the shameful sheep, Contessa the Controlling Cow, they can choose new responses. The responses naturally flow from this place of peace.

FEELING

Unloved		Unsafe	
Unloved	Inadequate	Powerless	Vulnerable
Unworthy	Unacceptable	Out of Control	Invalidated
Insignificant	Hopeless	Unsafe	Failure
Alone	Unwanted	Insecure	
Worthless	Disconnected	Devalued	
Unknown	Defective	Not Measuring Up	

COPING

BLAME	SHAME	CONTROL	ESCAPE
Blame others	Depressed	Perfectionistic	Drugs/Alcohol
Rage	Negative	Defensive	Numb Out
Angry	Anxious	Judging	Impulsive
Sarcastic	Inconsolable	Demanding	Video Games
Arrogant	Catastrophizing	Critical	Avoid Issues
Aggressive	Whine/Needy	Nagging	Hide Information
Discouraging	Manipulates	Lecture	Get Dramatic
Threatening	Withdraw to Pout	Withdraw to Defend	Act selfish
Hold Grudges	Isolate	Intellectualize	Minimizes
Retaliatory	Fault Finding	Controlling	Withdraw to Avoid
Withdraw to Punish	Shame Self		Irresponsible
Disrespectful			Escape

TRUTH

Loved	Accepted	Can Make Choices	Encouraged
Priceless	Promising	Precious	Connected
Treasured	Significant	Known	Can Control Self
Appreciated	Never Alone	Full of Worth	Wanted
Adequate	Valuable	Celebrated	

ACTIONS

Accepting	Non-Defensive	Energetic	Nurturing
Vulnerable	Hopeful	Supportive	Communicate Care
Respectful	Encouraging	Engaging	Open
Giving	Peaceful	Intimate	Welcoming
Let go/relax	Able to Persist	Kind	Settled
Responsible	Gentle	Seeking Good	Trustworthy
Listening	Forgiving	Honest	Listening
Merciful	Honest	Empathetic	Loving
Reliable	Humble	Valuing Self	Stay Connected
Inclusive	Positive	Self-controlled	Turn from Addictions

Figure 5.1 Feelings/Coping/Truth Actions Chart

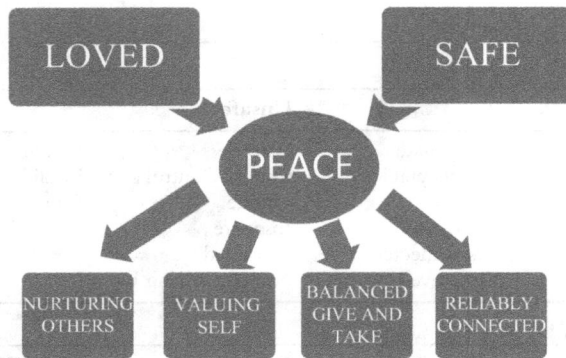

Figure 5.2 Peace Outflow

If we can help the child live out of the truth instead of what the Lying Lizard tells them about who they are. Rather than blaming, they can nurture others, rather than shaming themselves that can value themselves. Rather than overly controlling others or themselves, they learn to balance their relationships through partnership. Rather than escape, they can remain reliably connected.

Using the four coping characters the therapist can illustrate the transformation that takes place when kids settle into the truth. In this space of recognition, Brutus the Blaming Badger changes into Brutus the Boosting Badger (boosting and encouraging others rather than tearing them down.) Sharla the Shame Filled Sheep transforms into Sharla the Self-Assuring Sheep. Contessa the Controlling Cow turns into Contessa the Cooperating Cow. Eddie the Escape Goat changes into Eddie the Engaging Goat. The characters transform with the help of Shalom the Dove of Peace or Sammy the Sensible Squirrel (Wise-Selves). They tenaciously speak the truth to the coping characters, helping combat Lenny the Lying Lizard. Chapter 7 includes "session plans," which incorporate how to use these characters in helping children understand how they too can transform their troublesome behaviors.

The peace cycle also perpetuates further peace both with the self and others. The illustration below shows how this works. If a child is living out of their truth, it will positively impact other relationships.

After Stewart chose to believe the truth about himself, he entered into the Peace Cycle. Let's look at an example of Stewart's peace cycle:

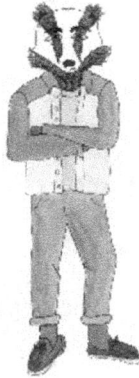

Figure 5.3 Brutus the Blaming Badger

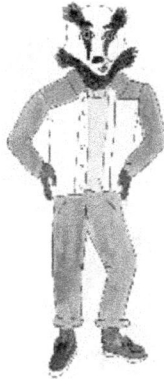

Figure 5.4 Brutus the Boosting Badger

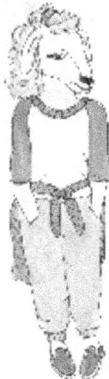

Figure 5.5 Sharla the Shame-Filled Sheep

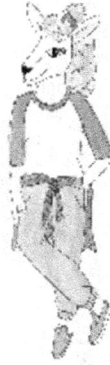

Figure 5.6 Sharla the Self-Assuring Sheep

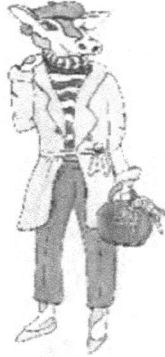

Figure 5.7 Contessa the Controlling Cow

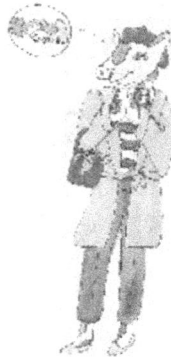

Figure 5.8 Contessa the Cooperating Cow

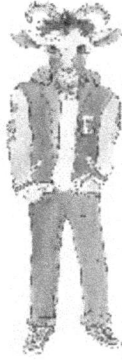

Figure 5.9 Eddie the Escape Goat

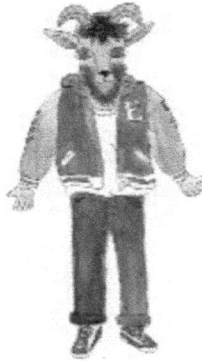

Figure 5.10 Eddie the Engaging Goat

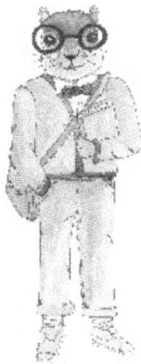

Figure 5.11 Sammy the Sensible Squirrel

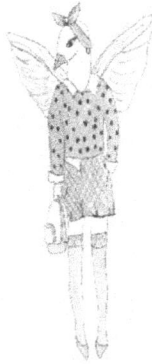

Figure 5.12 Shalom the Dove of Peace

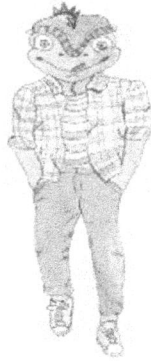

Figure 5.13 Lenny the Lying Lizard

Stewart's Truth:

1. He is loved
2. He is good enough
3. He is wanted

Stewart's Actions:

1. He values himself
2. He relaxed
3. He is joyful

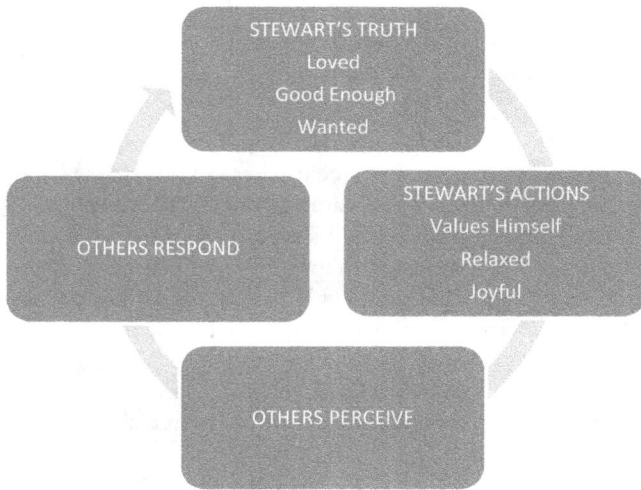

Figure 5.14 Stewart's Peace Cycle

It is helpful to write this out or to use the chart above. We can also use the pain and peace cards (with illustrations) to map this process out for children visually. Children, like adults, learn best in different ways. Some are more visually oriented, some are auditory learners and, others kinesthetic (Darling et al., 2014). I find it beneficial to get the brain involved in the session through various activities to help create new memories, primarily experiential memories of the peace cycle.

It is interesting to note that the latest brain research suggests that the labeling process or storytelling of our pain helps start to create positive change by employing our forebrain. Still, for trust to be developed and lasting peace to ensue, changes must be made through an experiential process (Hanna, 2014). This means that it is vital to lead the child through experiential exercises to help the peace cycle take root. For instance, the brain learns to trust much more quickly through things like "trust falls" than someone just telling me that they are trustworthy. Trust takes time and must be proven. Because of this, it imperative that a therapist is a trustworthy person, keeping a child's confidentiality at all costs, being consistently loving, reliable, and predictable in their responses, etc. . . . As a clinician, especially with children, our words are often less influential than our character.

Let's revisit our next session with Elise. We left off with her wanting to "pretend her Dad was sober." Let's observe an example of leading Elise into the peace cycle.

Next Session:

ELISE: Walks in and writes a 4.5 on the whiteboard, smiles, and sits on the couch.

THERAPIST: Hi, Elise! So, help me understand the 4.5.

ELISE: I'm not totally sure, but I am feeling less sad this week. I was just kind of like blah, but not terrible. I came out of my room more.

THERAPIST: Awesome! I am glad you stayed more connected, like the picture of the happily connected grapes we talked about a few weeks ago. So, you mentioned before you left last time that it might be a good idea to pretend Dad Goat is not drinking. Let's get the goats!!

ELISE: (laughing shyly) Okay!

THERAPIST: (puts Dad goat behind a pillow and takes him out again.) Okay, he is now sober. It is called "sober" when people are not drunk. Have you heard that before?

ELISE: Yes. I have heard my Mom say it, but I didn't know what it meant. He is sober. (Talking through daughter goat) Dad goat! I miss you when you are behind the pillow and acting weird, and you aren't sober. I barely see you on weeknights because you get home late, like at seven, and then I have to wash my goat hair and go to bed at 8:30 pm. On the weekends, you drink beer that tastes like pee, making you act mean and weird. I don't want to talk to you when you are like that.

THERAPIST: (talking now through Shalom the Dove of Peace) Oh wow, Edna! You have done a fantastic job of coming out of your room and talking to Dad Goat. I love how you waited to tell him this while he was sober and wasn't drinking. He can hear better then. I hear how you miss him and don't want him behind a pillow or a barrier. It is confusing because the drink doesn't look like a barrier, but it is.

ELISE: It is like a huge barrier!

THERAPIST: When people we love are not sober, we can feel sad, like homesick, or like we aren't even worth their time. It makes us wonder if they are safe to be around because the drink makes us feel unsure.
You did such a fantastic job of talking to Dad goat and letting him know what it feels like for you. Daughter goat! I think you deserve a blue ribbon at the fair because you have been brave and honest. Let's get you one!

ELISE: (speaking through Edna) Yay!! Thank you! Where do we go?

THERAPIST: (speaking through Shalom) Come with me and let's go to the fair where everyone can see you. Let's color a ribbon together. What should it say? How about something like I am known, I am empowered, I am connected. I'd like you to think of one of the best words while we make a ribbon. (Spend time together drawing, coloring, and creating a blue ribbon.)

ELISE: I think the daughter goat wants to be connected. Let's put that on the ribbon for her.

THERAPIST: I think that is a wonderful word. She is connected like you can be too.

ELISE: (grinning) Okay, let's tape this on Edna and take her into the arena at the fair.

THERAPIST: (Shalom hugs Edna) I am so proud of you! Daughter Goat You did such a great job trying to connect to your Dad and telling him how you feel instead of hiding in your room. Even though Dad Goat drinks sometimes, I want you to remind yourself of the truth that you can still connect with him when he is sober. You are connected to other people too. Who else are you connected to, like the happy little grapes in the picture?

ELISE: Oh, I always feel connected to my sister and brother and usually, my Mom! My grandma too! She is always there for me. She told me I could call her at midnight if I want.

Therapist (smiling) Do you feel safe with those people?

ELISE: Yes, for sure, all the time!

THERAPIST: Let's take Shalom and Edna and march around the arena (round coffee table) and repeat this together. "I am connected to a lot of safe people," "I am connected to a lot of safe people," "I am connected to a lot of safe people" (repeat at least ten times)

THERAPIST: Okay, that was such good work today. Let's put our puppets and toys away. Next time we will play some more and see how we can help Daughter Goat and Goat Dad.

I wonder what it might be like to talk to real Dad about drinking? (Says this while putting away toys indirectly and waits)

ELISE: Oh wow, nobody talks about Dad drinking, so I think that would be so scaaaaarrryy!!!

THERAPIST: Hmmm . . . Maybe it would be scary, and some things take a lot of courage. Daughter Goat was so brave when she reached out to connect to Dad Goat. I think she had some brilliant ideas about waiting to tell Dad Goat how she felt until he was sober.

Let's put these puppets back in their places and get Mom.

The therapist used Shalom the Dove of Peace's character to identify the truth and actions to help the client conceptualize a new way of relating and moving forward from pain to peace. It was an excellent way to help Elise process this. She was already naturally pressing toward change by imagining what it might look like for her to say something. The clinician was able to affirm this and use it as a launching pad.

The therapist identified the peace cycle by asking questions such as "what word is a good one to put on the ribbon for the fair?" The process of coloring this and writing out the word, followed by repetitive bilateral movements such as marching around the table, helps calm the mid-brain and experience a sense of peace. The verbal repetition of the peace cycle can prove very helpful for creating new neuro-pathways and enhance memory.

While children practice new patterns in our presence, we continue to use the "self" throughout the process by loving, affirming, and being a trustworthy presence. This helps children build the confidence necessary to break old patterns and step into new ones (Hanna, 2014).

References

Darling, C. A., Cassidy, D., & Powell, L. H. (2014). *Family life education: Working with families across the lifespan*. Waveland Press.

Feight, R. (2021). *Coping characters*.

Hanna, S. M. (2014). *The transparent brain in couple and family therapy: Mindful integrations with neuroscience*. Routledge.

Hargrave, S. (2011). *Building marriages for life and leadership*. The Hideaway Foundation.

Hargrave, T. D. (2019). *Advances and techniques in restoration therapy*. Routledge and Taylor & Francis Group.

Hargrave, T. D., & Pfitzer, F. (2011). *Restoration therapy: Understanding and guiding healing in marriage and family therapy*. Routledge.

Mellody, P. (1989). *Breaking free*. HarperCollins.

6 Bringing it Together

Practicing Mindfulness and the Four Steps

Along with any newly acquired skill-set, practice is required for it to become second nature. The four steps of moving from pain to peace in Restoration Therapy integrate many of the best practices of modern-day psychotherapeutic intervention and blend them into a practical and easy-to-remember strategy. These four steps help the child move from pain to peace within several minutes. As Restoration Therapy is experiential at its core, the therapist will execute the steps through an experiential approach using innovative play techniques and a song to help memorize the steps.

In taking a look at the next session, the clinician can observe what the process of moving out of pain into peace looks like in more depth. Additionally, this is a remarkable example of how a child can indeed affect the family system and propel the whole system toward positive change. In the following vignette, a top-down approach, where the parent was the first to be willing to make the change, would have been ideal, but it was not occurring due to alcoholism and codependence at the top of the family structure. Likely, because of the mother's codependent behaviors, she perpetuated the secrecy within the family and made it easier for Elise's Dad not to take responsibility for his actions (Mellody, 1989). In this powerful illustration, the reader will see how Elise, a nine-year-old girl, disrupted this painful familial cycle of relating.

Case studies like these help usher work with children forward under the umbrella of family therapy. It is easy to forget that children also have intrinsic power. As counseling seeks to empower them further, significant family change can and will occur. Nobody in the family system makes a change without a ripple effect. Even the smallest pebble thrown into a pond stirs the water, and the tiniest grains of sand act as purifying filters.

Elise' Next Session

THERAPIST: So, how is your overall mood this week? What is your number?

ELISE: My number is a 7 (smiling)

THERAPIST: (feigning falling over in the chair and popping up with a grin to match Elise's) A number 7!! It has never been that high before. Tell me what happened to cause it to climb 3.5 points!

DOI: 10.4324/9781003025504-6

ELISE: You are not even going to believe it!

THERAPIST: I can't wait to hear. (Leaning forward) I am literally on the edge of my seat. In fact, I am going to sit on the floor so I can hear you even better. (Sits on the floor.)

ELISE: (immediately flopping on the floor next to the therapist) Okay, well, I told my Dad that I wish that he would stop drinking. (a look of fear washed over her face.)

THERAPIST: Oh, my gosh! What did he do?

ELISE: Well, oh, my gosh is right! I was sooooo scared. He stopped looking at his phone and stared at me and just looked right in my eyes like this (drawing near and looking into the eyes of the therapist), and then he got up and left the room!

THERAPIST: Oh, wow! I can see how that might have made your heartbeat fast. Then what happened?

ELISE: Well, it did make my heart beat fast! I wanted to run to my room and cuddle with my cat, but I couldn't, or I would be like the sad, lonely grape in the picture (smiles), so I got up and followed him outside. He was cleaning the pool, and I cleared my throat really loudly like this (clears throat). Then I said, "Dad, are you mad at me?" He said he was not mad and said he hasn't drunk anything in a long time. (rolls her eyes) Well, I knew that wasn't true. I asked him about when he drank last weekend, and he fell asleep on the couch for like a whole day. I told him he was super grumpy too. He said he only drinks on the weekends, and then he tried to leave again! He started to go back into the house, and so I followed him again. I told him that is the only time I get to see him, and so it makes me feel really sad because he acts weird when he is drinking. I said sometimes he says mean things. He asked me about what weird things he did? I told him again that he says mean things too, like when he said he wished I had brown eyes like my Mom's. Then I started to cry a little bit. He came and hugged me and said he likes my eyes. When he said that, I started crying really hard like I was sobbing! I think this made my Dad feel sad, and he told me he loves me just the way that I am. He doesn't remember saying anything rude like that, and he said he was sorry.

THERAPIST: Oh, Elise! I hope you are so, so proud of yourself. I am happy that you said how you were feeling to your Dad. Do you know what I think you are? I think you are a truth-teller. It is just tremendous to be a truth-teller for other people and for ourselves, and you respectfully told the truth. Oh, my goodness, this is just great!! It can feel so scary, to tell the truth, but it also can feel really good in the end. I can hear you feel relieved, like there is a heavy blanket off of you.

ELISE: It does feel like that!! Oh, but I'm not finished talking.

THERAPIST: (chuckling) Go ahead. I want to hear every little bit of it!

ELISE: So then, like three days after that, I think it was Wednesday; my Dad said we were having a family meeting. My brother and I thought it was going to be about us doing our chores again. (frowns, then smiles) It was actually about my Dad starting to go to this meeting where he meets with other people, and they talk about sports and their health or something. (therapist smiles) Anyway, he is going every night, and at this meeting, they help each other not drink because they don't want to get fat, and beer can make you fat. Then you can't play sports. It is like a "get you in shape" meeting. My Dad isn't fat at all, but he likes sports a lot. It is called "Athletics A Must" or something like that.

THERAPIST: (hiding a grin) Hmmm . . . well, what do you think about Dad going to these meetings?

ELISE: Well, I am happy. He didn't drink at all this weekend!! I checked, and I couldn't find his beer anywhere. I looked in all of his hiding spots. There wasn't any beer behind the boat or in the shed.

THERAPIST: Wow!! Elise, I think your Dad listened to you, and it sounds like he is trying to stop drinking. It can be challenging for people to stop. Meetings with other people who are working to stop are really helpful. So, does it feel like you are in that arena with Daughter Goat? Why don't we get the puppets out?

ELISE: (smiles and scrambles to get the puppets, quickly grabs Daughter Goat, and starts walking her proudly about the room.)

THERAPIST: (talking through Dad Goat) Daughter Goat, thanks for talking to me. I am so glad you were brave and told me what you were thinking. My drinking doesn't have anything to do with you. It is hard for me to stop, but I am trying because I love you. I don't want to say mean things to you anymore. I think you are beautiful. I especially like your big blue eyes.

ELISE: (with Daughter Goat) Thanks, Dad Goat! I know. It is just that that gross drink makes me so sad and lonely, and I hope you don't do it again.

THERAPIST: (talking through Dad Goat) I am working not to right now.

ELISE: I know, Dad Goat. I Know. (hugging him)

THERAPIST: (getting the Shalom the Dove and speaking through Dove) Not all of the time but some of the time, people can start drinking again. I wonder what Daughter Goat might do if that would happen.

ELISE: I would talk to my Dad again when he isn't drinking and to my Mom. My Mom said I could tell her about it. They both said I could talk to you too, they said they wouldn't ask you or me what we said. Mom said she is proud of me for talking to my Dad, and she is sorry I felt like I couldn't talk to her. Also, I was thinking I could punch Dad in the face if he drinks again. (acts this out.)

THERAPIST: I can certainly understand how you would be angry Daughter Goat. It made you sad and hurt your feelings to think about that.

ELISE: I do want to beat up Dad Goat sometimes!! (continues to act out a fight and throwing Dad goat across the room.)

THERAPIST: Yes, Daughter Goat, you are so angry because you felt like you didn't know how to act when Dad Goat chose to drink over talking or being with you. It seemed like he wanted to drink instead of taking you ice-skating or to the daddy-daughter dance.

ELISE: (takes Daughter Goat and hides her behind a pillow pretends she is crying)

THERAPIST: What do we need to remember right now, Daughter Goat? What did we know and remember about who we are in the arena?

ELISE: That I am connected to a lot of safe people.

THERAPIST: (softens voice and speaks slowly through Shalom) Yes, we start feeling like we are alone, and we remember that we are connected to a lot of safe people. Let's say that together.

Say this with me:

"When I feel like I am alone, the truth is that I am connected."

(Therapist and Elise say this together five times.)

THERAPIST: So instead of hiding behind a pillow and getting very sad, what could you do, Daughter Goat? If you remember that you are Connected, how do you act?

ELISE: I come out from behind the pillow and talk to my Dad.

THERAPIST: So, you connect with your Dad and, if not your Dad, your Mom. You connect. Like the picture of the grapes (talk through peace cycle here)

ELISE: I love the connected grapes.

Moving to the Four Steps

THERAPIST: (through Shalom) I want to talk to you about the four steps. It is a perfect trick to help us when we start feeling sad. It is a great way to help us move from a 2 or 3 mood to an 8, 9, or even 10! after we practice it long enough, we can change our mood quickly. Can I tell you how to do the trick?

ELISE: (Jumping up and down) YES!!!!

THERAPIST: Okay. I am pretty excited to share this with you because it can help us feel so soo much better. Are you ready?

ELISE: Yes!!!

THERAPIST: Okay, so here goes. First, we will need to learn it and then we have to practice it a lot! Just like you practice your new dances for your shows. These are like learning new dance steps.

(Going to the whiteboard and writing down the following steps while speaking them aloud)

The Four Steps

Step 1. Say what I feel

Step 2. Say what I usually do

Step 3. Say the truth
Step 4. Say what I will do differently (Hargrave, 2019)

THERAPIST: I have a song that will help us remember, let's play it and try to learn it. Here are the words (hands Elise the lyrics and plays four steps song)

ELISE: I like that song!

THERAPIST: Yes, we will play it until we learn it really well. Can I ask you some questions first?

ELISE: Sure!

THERAPIST: So, when your Dad is drinking, what do you feel? (Now, the therapist writes the words Elise says next to the steps on the whiteboard.)

ELISE: When Dad drinks, I feel like the sad grape away from the rest of the bunch. I am alone.

THERAPIST: Perfect! That is step 1. When Dad drinks, I *feel* alone (writes it down). Okay, now, what do you usually do when you feel alone?

ELISE: When I feel alone, I go to my room.

THERAPIST: Okay, this is step 2. I usually go to my room or leave (writes it down)
What is the truth that we talked about? Are you truly alone like the grape?

ELISE: No, the truth is that I am connected to a lot of safe people!!

THERAPIST: AWESOME! You understand these steps! If you remember the truth, how do you act differently from what you act like in step 2?

ELISE: (smiling and waving her arm in the air to answer the question) I know it, I know it! I am brave and connect.

THERAPIST: You are correct; that is step four!! (writes it down) Okay, so now we can see your four steps! How about we read them together?

1. When Dad drinks, I feel alone
2. I usually would go to my room (avoid)
3. Instead, I am going to remember that I am connected to a lot of safe people
4. I will choose to be brave and connect

These are important steps to take, and if we can remember them and follow them. They *will* make us feel better.

ELISE: I think they will too!

THERAPIST: Let's get Edna Goat out and read the steps to her. Let's read them and say them to her five times while we sway back and forth like this. (Elise and Therapist practice repeating four steps together.) We are going to practice these steps every time you come in until they are impossible to forget! I hope you are so proud of your spectacular work this week and today! Do you want to erase the whiteboard while I put the puppets away? Or the other way around?

ELISE: I want to erase the board!

THERAPIST: Perfect, and then let's get Mom so we can schedule your next week.

The client continued to make wonderful progress over the next several months. Various methods were employed in working on the four steps. The four steps are the fourth and final objective of Restoration Play Therapy. After the client learns the four steps, it is necessary to continue encouraging the child to actively engage in the process when painful or conflictual events pop up. The therapist will continue to come alongside the client as a coach to help home in on each new skill that the four steps represent. The therapist takes the clients back to the process time and again until they are ready to move forward on their own. The following is a more detailed explanation of the four steps:

Objective Four: The Four Steps

Practicing the four steps rewires the brain and allows it to form new pathways (Hargrave, 2019). The steps were created to include much of the best and latest research. They are a concise way to walk the brain through mindfulness, emotional regulation, and CBT all at once. As was seen in the case study, the steps are as follows:

Step 1. Say what you feel
Step 2. Say what you usually do
Step 3. Say the truth
Step 4. Say what you will do differently

To effectively change previous maladaptive responses, a person has to validate their emotion, recognize their typical coping, remind themselves of a new truth then consciously make a new choice to respond differently. It is best to do this aloud as the brain typically moves onto new thoughts so quickly. When something is verbalized, it moves the information from the part of the brain that reacts to threat (the amygdala) to the part of the brain that engages in thought-based processes (the prefrontal cortex.) Repetition of this process will create new pathways in the brain. As the brain prefers what it is used to, it is imperative to practice, practice, practice, so the brain learns to prefer the peace cycle to the pain cycle (Hargrave & Pfitzer, 2011).

Step One: Say What You Feel

Moving from pain to peace and employing the four steps is easy to understand. The process can be executed sequentially. The patient first becomes aware of their painful feelings. Ideally, the clinician has explored this at length with them, and together they have precisely labeled the feeling words. This is a crucial step. Step One: Say what you feel. For years, science purported that thoughts trumped feelings. The reality is that *initially*, feelings trump a person's thoughts. They will win out every time (Siegal & Bryson, 2012). This is precisely why validating our painful emotion is the first order of business!

Validating our feelings allows the brain to begin to calm so that cognitive reasoning will follow. Feelings will never settle by ignoring them. It is utterly the opposite. Minimizing a child's emotions will inevitably result in them getting bigger and bigger until they are impossible to ignore. The energy that emotions produce will find a way to play out in one way or another. The hope is that they can be dealt with directly rather than being forced to come out sideways, in strange, destructive behaviors, or physiologically. When painful feelings are identified, they are automatically validated, and the midbrain immediately starts to settle (Siegal & Bryson, 2012). reality can be observed in very small children.

I was able to witness the positive reaction of emotional validation this past Thanksgiving. I had an opportunity to interact with a 13-month-old at a family gathering. She was quite upset that she was being thwarted from crawling backward down the staircase to yank the lamp cord from an out-let on the landing below her. She had managed to do it once, which had immediately gained the attention of three adults in the room, each calling her name and rushing toward her with concern.

She knew she mattered quite a lot in this instance. She did not respond in fear but instead grew a large four toothed grin. This is where the painful relational conflict began. She wanted the outlet and the attention. Mom wanted her safety. With the same rapidity she was removed with, she made a beeline straight back toward the prominent spotlight she had discovered.

Upon being scooped up by her Mom and carried up the stairs, she started to throw a baby fit. She arched her back while yanking her Mom's hair and began to fuss loudly. Mom held her and began to explain in a stern tone that the cord and outlet could hurt her. This brought on a litany of angry gib-berish, and her Mom loudly talked over her to logically explain the danger.

Instinctively knowing that emotional validation was needed to reach a teachable moment (Siegal & Bryson, 2012) and moved by compassion for them both, I sat down on the living room carpet and reached up toward the toddler, motioning her near. Mom put her down next to me while she continued to fuss loudly. I gently reached out to touch the arm of her little pink cardigan, which snugly outlined the many curves of her chubby arm. I rubbed her arm a moment, and she looked down with a curious frown. In a soft voice, I began. "I am so sorry that you feel sad and frustrated right now. It is hard to feel sad because you want to get the cord, and you can't." She sighed loudly, then quieted and immediately began to toddle off, which came as a bit of a surprise. A moment later, I observed her crouching in a struggle to pick up a picture book. With a concerted effort, she was able to grasp it precariously and moved back toward me, pivoting just as she was about to reach me. She backed herself up, tripped, and fell into my lap with her book. "Oh, thank you," I chuckled. Would you like to show me the pictures in your book? With this, she leaned with all of her tiny body mass into my chest, and I opened the book. She excitedly pointed to a dog. "What is that I asked?" "Pup-pup." She sighed and shook slightly as children often do when the energy of tears is released for good. Her Dad walked over and smiled. "Did you notice Pup-pup is to be said in a very distinct way? You inhale on the first pup and exhale with the last pup." We pointed to the dog again. Sure enough, Dad was correct, and we laughed.

We enjoyed the rest of the book while she popped her pacifier in and out of her mouth as we took turns talking about animal names, sounds, and colors. This example of helping give voice to a child's emotions underscores Step One: Say What you Feel. If a child cannot access the words, we make an educated guess and say the words for them. With good rapport established, kids are typically ready to correct the therapist if they don't quite have the right emotion. It is imperative to build good rapport at the onset of therapy as it is essential children feel very safe to give the therapist feedback.

Step Two: Say What You Usually Do

Second, the Step Two: Say What You Usually Do. This step helps slow down the impulsive reactivity and begins to engage the logical part of our brain. It might be appropriate to playfully tell a story about Lenny the Lying Lizard to help the child understand the need for Step Two. It would go something like this. "Because Lenny the Lying Lizard is cold-blooded, he is known to be exothermic. Can you say exothermic? Well, I wonder what exothermic might mean?" (allow them to guess.) "Hmmm . . . I like all of your ideas, they are outstanding, and I think you are good at figuring things out and being curious. Exothermic means that his environment controls his temperature. If he goes under a rock in the shade after a while, he will get too cold and will run really fast, like lightning" (move arms quickly back and forth in a running motion) "to get to a rock where he can lay in the sun. Then guess what happens when he realizes he is too hot?" (move arms quickly in a running motion again). "Can you move your arms like this? Yes, he panics, and his brain says," "I'm too hot!! I can't stand this!!!, I might die!!! I am afraid!!!" So, he obeys the feeling and runs, and if someone or another animal tries to stop him, what do you imagine he will do? (Allow for an answer) Yes! He will fight! He will act bigger and even do pushups to show he is strong! He will run at his opponent and will give some nasty bites! Sometimes our brain says the same kind of things to us. Sometimes or brain tells us we should run or fight. This is an excellent thing sometimes. I wonder when it might be a good thing and when it might not be a good thing? (Allow the child to answer and come up with various ideas.) Yes, I agree that would be good. When we are in real danger, our brains need to act fast, like lightning, so that we can move. Other times our brains need to remember that we aren't really in danger and that our feelings may be saying something that is not true. When this happens, instead of running or fighting, we can just stand our ground and take care of our hurting feelings. We are warm-blooded and not like Lenny, so we do not need to react to our environment in the same way. He lies to us sometimes, though, and makes us believe that we have to act just like him and get in a fight or run away to protect ourselves. But warm-blooded animals and people like us can choose to control and make good choices, no matter the environment around us. It just doesn't *feel* like that all the time. So, we need to say what we usually do after feeling hurt, scared or unloved in step two. In Step One, we give our feelings a name. In Step Two, we say what we usually do: Usually, I would run away, or usually, I would start a fight, or usually, I would say bad things about myself, or usually, I would boss my little sister around. This is Step Two. Say what you usually do.

Step Three: Say the Truth

In Step Three, the responsibility of the client is to access the truth. The therapist should have previously helped the client through the various ways to remind themselves of that which is true. People can access the truth about their safety and identity from others, themselves, faith sources. Steps one and two have helped calmed the brain enough for the brain to access logical thought, and the brain is primed to be soothed. In Step Three, we can simply encourage the child to step into the first part of the peace cycle by reminding themselves to challenge their painful feelings with positive reality. The truth sounds like this: I am loved, I have the power to choose, I am treasured, I am important, I am strong, I can persevere. It may even be helpful to access all three of the truth resources after completing Steps One and Two. For instance, Step One: I feel unwanted, Step Two: Usually, when I feel unwanted, I would start bragging about myself. Step Three: The truth is that I am wanted by my oldest sister, my dog, my teacher, Mrs. Miller. I also know that God made me just like he wanted me to be, and he wants me. I also believe I am worth being wanted. I am a good friend and fun to be around. This example illustrates how the child accessed the truth from others, his faith, and himself. Step Three is also imperative to practice often with the child to be assured there is a firm knowledge of how to move forward.

Step Four: Say What You Will Do Differently

During this final step, the child's mind and body are feeling much more settled. If they do not appear or feel more at peace, encourage them to continue to meditate on Step Three until they start experiencing these changes. From this stable place, prompt them to verbalize what they are going to do differently. It may prove helpful to revisit Step Two, Say: What You Used to Do. Step Four is typically an antithetical action. For example, if the child says: "When I feel unsafe at night, I run to my Mom and Dad's bed to sleep. Instead, they can say: "The truth is that I am safe in my bed, and so I will stay here. The four steps would go as follows:

1. Say What You Feel: I feel unsafe
2. Say What You Do: When I feel unsafe I, usually run to my Mom and Dad's bed
3. Say the Truth: The truth is that I am safe. My Mom and Dad told me that they locked the doors and a robber has never broken into our house. God is strong and able to protect me. I can pray and ask God to protect me. I can choose to trust Mom and Dad. I can choose if I did really see a robber to call for help. I can call my parents or call 911 with my cell phone. I don't see a robber. I am safe at this moment.
4. Say What You Will Do Differently: I will stay in my own bed and go to sleep on my own. I don't need to get in trouble because the house is safe right now.

The Four Steps are an effective strategy, employing mindfulness, CBT, and emotional regulation. The following is an innovative song and pneumonic device to help kids practice and repeat the steps to moving from pain to peace.

Four steps

Pain to Peace Song Lyrics

by Micah John Frigaard

Step 1,2,3 4
when my heart is sore
I know the way
to help me feel better

Step 1 I say what I feel down in our heart,
Then say what I used to do, yeah that's the 2nd part
Then 3 sets me free; I tell myself the truth.
Then step 4 comes simply, change my actions. There's your proof

The proof to changing your pain to peace these are the easy steps that you can achieve

Step 1,2,3 4
when my heart is sore

I know the way
to make me feel better

Step 1,2,3 4
when my heart is sore
I know the way
to make me feel better
make me feel better
better

References

Hargrave, T. D. (2019). *Advances and techniques in restoration therapy*. Routledge and Taylor & Francis Group.

Hargrave, T. D., & Pfitzer, F. (2011). *Restoration therapy: Understanding and guiding healing in marriage and family therapy*. Routledge.

Mellody, P. (1989). *Breaking free*. HarperCollins.

Siegal, D. J., & Bryson, T. P. (2012). *The whole-brain child: 12 Revolutionary strategies to nurture your child's developing mind*. *Bantam books trade PBK*. New York: Bantam Books

7 Session Plans and Practical Tips for Therapists

We have talked about therapy being both an art and a science. The following part of this book is going to give a framework to the art. Like the best sort of poetry, RT has a great structure to work within creatively. If we lean too heavily on the structure, there is a risk of the child feeling too controlled or moving too quickly through the therapeutic plan's steps and objectives. Conversely, if we have no form or structure and lean too heavily on the creative side, things can feel confusing and boundaryless for both child and therapist. The key is to blend the two.

The following session plans are best maneuvered through in fluid form. Please weave in your creative ideas as they surface. Feel just as free to listen to the child when they have a clever idea they want to try out. We do want to direct the session back to the treatment objectives. However, there is much room for freedom within the boundaries. After all, only with boundaries can we genuinely understand and attain true freedom. Let's model this practice with kids.

As Julie Andrews touted in her endeavor to teach music to the Von Trapp children, "the very beginning is a very good place to start." In supervising new therapists, I am consistently reminded that what to do in the very first session is a great place to begin. The following session plans can be implemented in order and sequential practice, or they can be used in ways that make sense to what the child is facing at the particular time. You need to use discretion to apply the following ideas for what is pertinent to the client's need.

These ideas may also be applied to adult clients with some adaptation. The saying "a picture is worth a thousand words" is correct. The object lessons and illustrations in the following session plans have proven invaluable to adults in the healing of their inner-child or reparenting practices.

These session plans are structured similarly to educational lesson plans for teachers. The session plans provide creative ideas while helping. We guide the child toward the treatment objective. When making brain changes, the brain responds most effectively to novelty and familiarity. The plans follow a similar structure but vary in theme. This provides children with a sense of what to expect, which translates into safety.

The main two themes of reaching emotional peace in the work of Restoration Therapy are love and safety. Therefore, the main two goals in

DOI: 10.4324/9781003025504-7

implementing the session plans are to implement them with a genuine love for the child while providing safety and trustworthiness. Under these overarching themes, we will be able to employ the self as a change agent in many children's lives. It is agreed that parents are the original brain programmers. Many Dads throw their kids in the water to teach them how not to drown. However, it is often the swim coach who helps that same child hone their skills. They help children rid themselves of ineffective movements and replace them with efficient strokes to skim across the water and into huge wins they may never otherwise experience. Guiding children in helping rewire troublesome and painful neuro pathways is a worthy and joyful endeavor. We hope that each therapist finds much joy and fulfillment in the practice of helping many children play their way from pain to peace and move forward with practical tools that will last them a lifetime.

Restoration Therapy Session Plans for Kids—Overview

Restoration Therapy revolves around four steps.

*   Identifying **pain**
*   Acknowledging **coping** habits
*   Discovering the **truth**
*   Determining **action** (behavioral change based on that truth)

In adapting these steps to children, we will constantly be building rapport, so we have added that as Step Zero. The whole process will look like this:

0. Building rapport—
1. Identifying **Pain**ful feelings

    a. Unloved
    b. Unsafe

2. Identifying **Coping**

    a. Shame
    b. Blame
    c. Control
    d. Escape

3. Discovering the **Truth**—These experiential activities help the child learn and experience in session what the truth about them actually is.
4. Changing our **Actions**—These activities help the child identify and practice taking different action steps

The therapist can determine which step the child is working on (Steps Zero to Four) and match it with a helpful session plan by noting the "Restoration Therapy Steps," These appear at the beginning of each session plan.

The First Session

Restoration Therapy Steps Zero to Two
Age Level: 4 to 18
Materials Needed:

- Prepared Lobby
- Practices Intake Paperwork
- Inside Out Emotion figurines.

Treatment Objectives (Purpose):

- Begin building rapport
- Help child and parents to understand counseling process, paperwork, confidentiality
- Assess needs for diagnostic impression and treatment goals

Buy-in and Focus: Building Rapport

Rapport begins in the lobby; ensure your lobby has something inviting to children in it, a little table with coloring books, toys, a candy dish, pictures that will allow a child to know they are welcomed and belong. When greeting a parent and child, greet the parent first. This allows the child to observe your warm interaction with their parent or guardian first, without immediately being put on the spot. Then turn to the child and, if possible, crouch down to their level and smile. "Hello there, my name is Ms. Nancy. I am so glad to meet you. Thank you so much for coming to visit me today. Let's see where my office is. Mom or Dad, let me have you lead. Go ahead down the hall to the last door on the right." (Follow the family and as they enter the room, let them know they can sit wherever they would like.)

Thank you again for coming! It looks like you have filled out your paperwork, so let me just take a minute to look this over. Quickly skim paperwork to ensure all is complete. Give careful attention to signatures. State the Objectives.

Understanding Counseling Process: *So, first, I would like to ask* (child's name) *what he/she has heard about counseling. It can sometimes be confusing, so I wonder what you might think people do in counseling?* (Allow the child to answer.) Some will know. Often, they will not. Try to find something about their answer to agree with or at least smile at. Thank them for answering the question and their good idea.

Yes, so coming to see a counselor is a little bit like going to a doctor, but we don't give anybody medicine or shots or anything like that here. We aren't doctors for hurt bodies. We are like doctors or nurses for hurting emotions. (Now, point to the Inside-Out Emotion figurines.) *These are some emotions; maybe you have seen this movie? Can you pick up one of those emotions and tell me his name?* Do this one by one and help if needed. *So, I wonder if we think any of these emotions good or bad?* (Allow the child to answer) typically they will let you know that "Joy" is the only good one. *Hmmm . . . Joy is the one that feels good, huh? You are right about that, but actually, they are all good because they each have an important job to do. Take the Fear figurine in your hand. "This is good too. Do you know why? Well, let's see . . . what if Spiderman was our friend and he scooped us up and set us on top of a huuuuge tall building, and the building started to shake. If we didn't have web powers like Spiderman, we would feel very afraid. So that "afraid feeling" would tell us to take care of ourselves. How might we take care of ourselves in that situation?*

Yes! We would back up from the edge of the building and use our loud voice to ask for help and say, "Hey Spiderman! I need some help here!! If we didn't have that feeling of fear, we wouldn't know or care to do that. So, fear is a good thing in that situation. All of these emotions tell us something really important. We will talk more about them later.

When we hurt our bodies, like fall down on our bikes and get a big scrape, it usually has dirt in it or rocks or something. What do we need to do to take care of our hurts? Yes, we need to clean it out and then put a band-aid on it, or if it is broken, a cast. Talking about our hurt feelings is exactly a way to clean them out so they can start to heal and feel better! I really want to help people feel better, and I am pretty good at it because I do it every day. I have learned about the best ways to help. So, we will do a lot of talking in here and playing, drawing, and pretending too!

Paperwork/Confidentiality: Return attention to paperwork. *Our paperwork talks about several things; I want to take a moment to talk about confidentiality.* (Ask child) *Do you know what the word confidentiality is? It is a big word.* (Allow for an answer). *Yeah, it can be hard to understand. Confidentiality means that I will not talk to other people about what we talk about in here. It will stay private. I won't tell your friends, or teachers, or even your parents about what we say in here unless it has to do with keeping you safe. If, for some reason, you aren't safe. I will need to talk to another adult about that. Like if someone were hurting you or you were somehow going to be unsafe. Other than that, I think it is really important that you can say whatever you want in here and I won't tell anyone.* (Smiling) *Now, you can talk to people like your parents about what we talk about here. The only deal I am making is that I won't say anything. It would be weird if an adult ever asked you not to talk about something or keep it a secret. That is weird, so you are free to talk to other people. Does that make sense?* (check for understanding.)

Turn to Mom and Dad. *So, Mom and Dad, in my work, I have found this to be important. If a kid thinks I will tattle on them, then good trust can't be built. This space can help kids talk about whatever they need to talk about without feeling like they might get in trouble for it. Sometimes they may be confused, mad, or frustrated with their parents, just like we were as kids. It can be so relieving to have another adult to talk through these things with. Also, as a family therapist, I very much encourage inviting you in at the beginning or end of the session to sit with your child so we can talk about anything that can be helpful. When we talk together, they know I am not going behind their back. I will encourage your child to be as open as possible with you because you are typically their biggest advocate, and the goal is not to be in therapy forever. I will let your child take the lead in these check-ins and encourage them to bring up things I think will help the healing process. It may take a little bit before we figure out what is most helpful for them to talk through. Does that all sound okay with you? Do you have any questions about the paperwork or confidentiality? Great. Sessions typically last about 50 minutes. Oh, and also, if you do need to cancel, please let me know 24 hours in advance; that would be great. Otherwise, the office will charge the session fee.*

Assess Needs/Diagnostic Impression/Treatment Goals. Ask the parents; *I would like to know some of the things that you like about your child. What are some of their strengths?* This question helps build rapport with all parties and gives us a first look into what the "truths" and the peace cycle may be for this child. *Ahhh . . . these are wonderful things. I can't wait to know more about your son or daughter; he/she sounds amazing!*

Can you tell me what the reason is that you decided to bring (name of child) in to get some help? Listen to see what the possible pain cycle may be. Are the parents mentioning painful feelings the child has talked about or troublesome ways they are coping? *Hmmm . . . it sounds like there is a lot going on.* (reflect an understanding of the main issues and ask for clarification.) *Hmm . . . yes, that makes sense, and I am happy to help. This does sound painful.*

What things would you most like to see change for (name of the child?) (Here, we are searching to hear what the goals are and reiterating them for clarification.) *So, to clarify, (Child's Name) is experiencing anxiety in school and having difficulty feeling peaceful while separated from the family. You would like him to be able to go to school without worrying so much?* If affirmed, continue. *How long has this been going on? Is it worsening or getting better? Has anything happened like this in the past? Have there been any recent possibly upsetting events or changes in his/her environment?* Continue to ask the questions on the assessment.

When finished, thank the family for coming in. *It was very nice to meet you all. Mom and Dad, if you would like to wait in the lobby (Child's Name), I will meet for the rest of the session.* Stand up and open the door for Mom, Dad, or Guardian.

Pick one of the preliminary shorter activities to assess painful feelings or coping—Perhaps the Adapted Kinetic Drawing.

Session Summary: Thank the child for their participation. *Super job, it has been so nice to meet you. Thank you for all of your good work. Let's pick up these toys and then go get Mom/Dad in the lobby.* (After thanking them for picking up the toys, travel with them to the lobby.) *Hey Mom and Dad! Go ahead and come on back.*

After everyone is seated once again, *I appreciate you coming in, and I think there is some good work to be done to help (Child's Name) start to feel some relief. Thank you for (loosely restate the first session objective) for letting me get to know you a little bit and allowing me to explain the counseling process. I have all of your paperwork, and we have a couple of goals written down. Would you like to set up a follow-up appointment now, or would you rather give me a call to set something up?*

Sounds good; let me just check my calendar. It looks like I have some availability next week on Tuesday at 2 pm. Does that work? Alright, I will schedule it right now and look forward to seeing you then. Standing up, address the child directly. *Again, it was so very nice to meet you, and I will see you soon. Have a good week!* Open the door and direct them toward the exit.

Adapted Kinetic Drawing

Restoration Therapy Steps One to Two
Age Level: 4 to 18
Materials Needed: Blank paper, markers, crayons, pencils.
Treatment Objective (Purpose): Identify conflict within the family system, painful feelings, and coping methods. (blame, shame, control, escape.) Activity: The Client will create a drawing of their family in a conflict.

Buy in and Focus—Thank the child for coming into your office and prompt them to sit on the floor with you. Mirror their body language. After they get comfortable, ask: *What was one good thing that happened this week? What was one hard thing?* Reflect what you heard and mirror their emotion when reiterating both stories. *Hmmm . . . The hard thing does sound hard; thank you for sharing that with me. Is there anything else? Ahhh. Thank you for sharing that too.* Sometimes it helps to draw pictures. *I would like us to draw a picture.*

Psychoeducation: *I would like us to remember a time when we were in an argument or upset at our family or someone in our family. Include everyone in your family in a drawing doing something while this argument or disagreement was happening. Then afterward, I would like to talk about it.*

Modeling (show): Direct the child to blank paper and markers, pencils, crayons. Allow the child the decision of which writing tool to use.

Intervention (practice alongside): Come alongside the child with encouragement for participating and occasionally prompt the child during the drawing reminding the child to ensure each family member is present in the picture and needs to be doing something, but they get to choose what that is. Allow the child space and quiet to complete the drawing.

Checking for Understanding: After the child completes drawing, compliment them on their work and ask the following questions while being careful to reflect their answers:

1. *"Can you tell me the names of everyone in the picture?"*
2. *"Tell me about what is happening in the picture."*
3. *"What sorts of things are you feeling right now in this picture?"*
4. *"What are you doing in the picture?"*
5. *"What do you wish you could do instead of what you are doing in this picture?"*
6. *"Tell me what Mom, Dad, Sister, Brother, Dog are doing in the picture?"*

7. *"Is there anything else you would like to tell me about this picture?"*
8. *"Do you feel like I understand it all pretty well?"*

Individual (Brain-Changing) Practice: *Wow! you did such a great job talking through that. I really do feel like I can picture what was happening. Can you tell me again maybe three feelings you were having during this argument?* Repeat their painful feeling words to the child. *Now, can you tell me what you usually do when you feel this way?* (listen for coping words and assess for overarching themes of blame, shame, control, or escape.)

  Session Summary *Wow! Awesome. I think you did very well, telling me about some painful feelings and what you do with those sometimes. I like this picture because it helps me to get to know you better. I can already tell you are such a (loveable) kid.* (try to use the opposite word as one of the child's stated painful feeling words. If a child felt "unloved" during the argument, use the words "loveable" or "important.") *You helped me understand that sometimes when we are in an argument or something hard is going on; we can feel (state expressed feeling words.) That is hard to feel that way, and so when we start to feel those things, we might want to (state coping words here.) It makes sense. Also, it makes sense we could get into trouble or feel worse when we do those things. Hmmm . . . How about we start to figure out how we can start feeling better? Okay, great. Let's put these papers and writing things away and go get your Mom and Dad. Thanks so much!!*

Lenny the Lying Lizard

Restoration Therapy Steps Zero to Two
Age Level: 5–16
Treatment Objective (Purpose): The child will be able to identify
  and define the painful feeling and explain how they lead to the fight
  or flight response
Materials: Squishy lizards, picture of Lenny the Lying Lizard and Sammy,
  the Sensible Squirrel.

Buy in and Focus: Welcome the child into the office and sit on the floor with them. Bring out squishy lizard toys and toss one to them. (Allow the child to handle and play with the lizard for a while. Invite the child to toss him back and forth like a ball while asking questions.) *How was your week? Was there anything fun that you did? Was there anything hard that happened when you started to feel bad again? Tell me about that.* (Reflect their narrative and mirror their emotions.) *Hmmm . . . that does sound hard. So, I would like to tell you something about lizards. What do you know about Lizards?* (Let them reply.) *Yes, I can see you know some good things about lizards. I am going to tell you something else that is good to know about them. First, though, let's do something together.*

  Let's stand up and put our arms straight out to the side. Okay, now we are going to make our hands into fists, and we will make arm circles like this. Okay, but first, let's stop for a second, and I will time us and see how long we can go. (Set timer) *On your mark, get set, go!* (make arm circles together for as long as you can. As you see, child tiring let them win and stop the clock when they drop their arms. Write down the time on a whiteboard or a piece of paper.) *Good job!! Okay, let's sit down, and I would like to tell you about this Lizard.* Show them a picture of Lenny the Lying Lizard.

Psychoeducation: *Okay, so I am going to tell you a secret that may be good to remember for your whole life. We all have a little lizard-like Lenny who lives in our brain* (referring to the reptilian part of our brain that induces fight or flight), *and when we get upset about something, like the hard thing we talked about that happened this week. Lenny gets really uncomfortable. You see lizards absorb the environment around them. They cannot control (regulate) their own temperature because they are cold-blooded. This is why Lenny has to sit on warm rocks when it gets too cold or when it gets too hot; he has to run in a cooler hole or away from the heat. If it is too hot or cold, he can't stand it, and so he starts to tell us lies sometimes so that we will fight or run to try and get our uncomfortable situation will stop. Does that make sense?*

Modeling (show): *Okay, let's put Lenny on the top of the table under the lamp. Oh!! He is getting uncomfortable. What is he going to do? Yes! he is going to run away and find a cool spot. Now let's put him in a cool spot like under this couch cushion.* (instruct the child to act like a freezing wind and blow in Lenny's direction.) *Oh, my goodness, he is peeking out, and I can see he is getting very cold, but he is scared to get past you, but if he doesn't come out, he is afraid he might die. So be careful, he is going to fight his way out of there, and he may bite you on the nose. He is trying to survive!!*

Sometimes, he does help us try to survive, but a lot of times, he tells us lies because, unlike him, we have a superpower. Do you know what it is? We can regulate our own body temperature. It takes some practice, but we can do it. Because we also in our brains have Sammy, the Sensible squirrel who is the boss of Lenny. Here is Sammy's picture.

(Show the child the picture and let them know we will talk more about him later.) *Okay, let's try something, and I want us to try to hear Lenny and Sammy talking to us.*

Intervention (practice alongside): *Now, we will try and beat our time doing the arm circles. Be ready because we will get tired and want to stop, and when that happens, I want us to listen for Lenny the Lying Lizard's voice. He is going to say things, like, "You can't keep this up. You are too weak! Your arms are going to fall off! You need to stop now!" He will say some other things, too; let's both listen to what he says. But then I also want us to listen to Sammy, the sensible squirrel who will tell us the truth. He will encourage us and say, "You are strong." "You can do this!" "You did it before, and you can go a little longer." "Your arms are not going to fall off."*

Checking for Understanding: *Okay, are you ready? Tell me what we are going to do right now after we set the timer. Who are we going to listen for, and what might they say?*

Individual (Brain-Changing) Practice: Set the timer and begin to do arm circles. Feel free to invite the child to yell out messages they hear with prompts like: *What is Lenny the Lying Lizard saying right now? What is Sammy saying that is the truth? Who is going to win? Let's beat that timer!!*

Session Summary: *Great job beating that timer! You listened to the truth!* If the child doesn't beat the timer, let him know we will try next time and that it is okay. Talk through feelings and identify reasons they weren't able to believe they could do it. Validate emotions. *So, this is like our feelings when we are experiencing something difficult. Perhaps like a disagreement with Mom and Dad. Lenny might start yelling at us and tell us that we are (one of the child's identified pain words) "unloved." He wants us to do something to scramble away from that feeling or to have us bite somebody on the nose. He lies and says this will make the feeling go away forever. But what do you think the truth is? What is something Sammy, who is the truth part of our brain, might tell us?* (Allow the child to answer and clarify and guide as needed.) *Good job! Sammy helps us to remember that we are loved. You did such good work today. I can't wait to talk more next week. Let's pick up these toys and go and get Mom and Dad.*

Sammy The Sensible Squirrel and the Shalom the Peaceful Dove

Restoration Therapy Steps Three to Four
Age Level: 5 to 16
Materials: People puppets, Lenny the Lying Lizard, Sammy the Sensible Squirrel, Shalom the Dove of Peace.

Treatment Objective (Purpose): The child will identify the power of the Wise-Self through understanding that they have a choice to talk to their painful feelings sensibly and subsequently experience peace. The child will imagine and practice implementing voices of the Wise-Self.

Buy in and Focus Welcome child warmly and invite them to sit down with you on the floor. Grab Lenny the Lizard and began to toss him back and forth.) *So, do you remember this guy? What is his name, and what does he do?* (Allow the child to answer.) *Great job.* (Clarify if needed.) *So, I wonder if we heard him whispering to us this week? Did we feel upset about something, in particular, that happened? Tell me about it. Hmmm . . . so I agree those thoughts are just like things Lenny the Lying Lizard may tell us. He is pretty rotten. So, today I would like us to meet someone else.*

I want us to meet a squirrel and a bird today. (Show the puppets or a drawing of them to the child.) *This is Sammy the Sensible Squirrel, and this is Shalom the Dove. Do you know what the word "Shalom" means? It means peace or harmony, like when everything is just like it should be, and we can just lay down and sigh and say, "ahhhhh . . ." I am not afraid or scared, I feel loved and important and protected. I am not worried about anything. I wonder if you have ever felt that way before. What is a time you can remember when you felt peace like that?* (Allow the child to answer, and as they answer, be listening for words that will likely be a part of their specific peace cycle.) *Oh, my goodness! That sounds wonderful! So, Sammy the Sensible Squirrel and Shalom the Dove want to help us experience this feeling of peace when Lenny, the lying Lizard, lies to us and tells us mean things.*

Psychoeducation: *You know when you told me about when* (use child's own painful story they have told you) *your Mom and Dad told you they were going to get a divorce? I remember you said you were so sad, and you were worried that you did something wrong to make them get a divorce. You said you felt like they didn't love you anymore and that nothing would be the same anymore, and you felt scared. So, it sounds like you felt guilty, unloved, and afraid. Is that right?* (wait for clarification and clarify pain words until there is a good understanding of the child's painful feelings. Allow plenty of time to pinpoint correct feelings and speak gently, curiously, and in nurturing tones when questioning the child.) So, guilty, unloved, and afraid. Hmmm . . .

Modeling (Show): *I would like you to grab a puppet that looks like you or a puppet you would like to pretend is you. Great job, that puppet does remind me of you!* With Lenny, the Lying Lizard in hand and a "lizard voice," repeat the child's pain words to the puppet. "*Guilty, unloved, afraid . . . nothing will ever be the same.*" Oh wow! Those are really painful things for Lenny to say, and really, they are not true! Those are lies. We need some help here! (Pretend Sammy the Squirrel and Shalom the Dove are running and flying to the scene.) *Speaking through Sammy, the Squirrel puppet say, "Lenny, get out of here! Are you telling your big fat lies again? You need to stop doing that. (Child's Name) is not like you. His environment doesn't control him. You are cold-blooded; he is warm-blooded. He can make choices about telling himself the truth and choices about his actions and start to feel better."* (Give Shalom the Dove puppet to the Child and instruct the child to start telling the truth to the puppet representing him.

Intervention (practice alongside): Come alongside the child. *What is your puppet believing about himself right now when his parents just told him they were getting a divorce?* (allow for an answer, listening for pain words.) *Okay, so he is believing Lenny the Lying Lizard's words right now.* (Hand the child Shalom the Dove.) *Now, have Shalom tell him* (pointing to the child's puppet) *what is true. What does your puppet need to hear right now?* (allow answer, taking note of peace words. Help child to identify the accurate words.) *Great job. Shalom told your puppet he needed to know the truth is that this divorce is not his fault. He is innocent. His parents still love him, and so do a lot of other people. Not EVERYTHING is going to change, just some things, and he will still be safe. So, Shalom just told your puppet that you are innocent* (not your fault), *loved, and safe.* (Picking up Sammy the Sensible Squirrel and speaking through him.) *I agree you are innocent, loved, and safe. When you hear me say that, how do you feel?* (Allow the child to answer through his puppet.)

Checking for Understanding: *So, can I ask you something? When something hard happens, like when our parents tell us they are getting a divorce, what are some things Lenny the Lying Lizard might tell a kid?* (Allow time to answer.) *Yes, he shouts painful emotions at us. What should we do when we start to feel those things? Correct, we need to listen for another voice like Sammy's or Shalom's. What do Sammy and Shalom tell us? Yes, they tell us the truth, and then how do we feel? Absolutely, we feel happier and peaceful and then make better decisions. Do you think we only need to tell Lenny one time to be quiet and listen to Sammy or Shalom? You* *are correct; the answer is no. We have to practice this over and over and over again! Let's practice again right now.*

Individual (Brain-Changing) Practice

So, let's pretend that somebody tells your puppet this week that Dad might go on a fun vacation with his new wife and her kids while you are staying at Mom's. Go ahead and pick up Lenny the Lying Lizard and tell me what he might say to your puppet. (Allow the child to answer. Speak slowly and show empathy while you help the child express painful feelings.) *Now, I think Lenny is telling mean lies again! Go ahead and pick up Shalom. What do you think Shalom is going to say to your puppet? Lenny told your puppet that he was unloved and unsafe, that Dad might like his step-kid more now. Let Shalom tell your puppet what he needs to hear.* (Allow the child time to state and practice his truth words.)

Session Summary *Wow. Such a great job today. We learned a lot about how Lenny the Lying Lizard isn't the boss of us. We learned that we can say our painful feelings and can ask the Shalom part of our brain to talk to the painful feeling part of our brain. You can keep practicing this all week. I would like to hear next week how it goes! Let's pick up our toys and go get Mom and Dad.*

Coping Characters

Blame, Shame, Control, and Escape
Restoration Therapy Step Two
Age Level: 5 to 16
Materials Needed: Four Coping Character Puppets, RT for Kid's Song
download.
Treatment Objective: The child will define and identify four coping characters, which represent blame, shame, control, and escape. The child will recognize personal coping methods when experiencing emotional pain.

Buy in and Focus: Warmly welcome and invite patient to have a seat on the floor. *How was your week? What was something good that happened and something hard that happened?* (Reflect empathy and validate feelings.) *How did you respond when this happened?* (Observe from stated response how the client may be coping, what are the unhelpful responses?) *Thank you for sharing that. I have some animals that I would like you to meet today. Let me get them.* (Retrieve puppets.)

Psychoeducation: *These puppets are important because they help us understand what we do when our feelings are hurting. So, let's say a kid at school told us that we were wearing a really ugly outfit and looked stupid. What might we do if that happened? Do you think we would just sit there and smile? No, probably not. We would react. These animals would all react, but they have different reactions. I wonder* *why we might react?* (Let the child answer.) *Oh, you are so smart! I agree; yes, we want it to stop happening because it is hurting us. Somehow our reaction is trying to protect us. You have such good answers.*

Modeling (Show): *First, I want to show you this guy. Do you know what animal he is? You are right! He is a badger, and his name is Brutus the Blaming Badger. Okay, I want you to remember these animals' names because I'll ask you at the end of the session. So, this is Brutus the Blaming Badger. This is Sharla, the Shame-Filled Sheep. This is Eddie the Escape Goat, and this is Contessa, the Controlling Cow. Whenever any of us has a sore or hurt feeling, we react. So, like the kid who said our outfit is ugly or if our brother or sister called us a mean name, we all react. It is just sometimes we react in ways that get us into trouble. These four guys get themselves into trouble a lot by how they cope with having a sore feeling. As I talk through how they act when they are hurt, I'd like you to think about which one or two you are most like.*

Intervention (practice alongside): Lead the patient through an interactive introduction to the puppets.) *Hi, I am Brutus, and if someone does something rude. I am rude back! I sometimes yell really loud, and if someone says I am stupid, I just say, "No, I AM NOT!! YOU ARE ACTUALLY THE STUPID ONE!" I start to stand up super tall and puff my chest out and argue. Sometimes I get in trouble at school for fighting, and I get so angry!! I tell people everything is their fault and the reason I am yelling is because of you and what you did.*

Hi. I am Sharla the Shame-Filled Sheep. If someone tells me I am stupid or ugly, I want to shrivel up like a little dumb raisin and disappear. I get so embarrassed and think that they are probably right, and I wonder why I ever decided to wear this stupid outfit. If I just get really quiet and don't say or do dumb things anymore, maybe it will be better. I feel really sad a lot and feel worthless or like a piece of trash that somebody should pick up and throw away.

Hi. I am Contessa, the Controlling Cow. First of all, people probably won't say I dress dumb because I don't. I plan out all of my outfits and make sure they are ironed and don't have any wrinkles, and I would never wear anything ugly. If someone thought that, I would show them how expensive my outfit is and let them know I have checked all the fashion magazines and probably learn what is in style because I know it all. I know almost everything there is to know. I work hard, and I like to tell other people what to do. If they don't want to listen or be helpful, I will just do it myself because I don't trust other people to know what they are talking about. I can do everything the best. I would wonder why this little peasant is talking to me about nice clothes because they don't have a clue!! I am not afraid to tell them that too. Other animals are so ridiculous.

Hi, I am Eddie, the Escape Goat. I just want to get along with people, and if someone was rude and told me my outfit was ugly. I would probably just shrug and walk away. I don't like fighting. I would feel bad inside, but I will deal with it on my own. When I start to remember the mean things they said, I will do something else like play a video game or daydream or feel numb inside if people say mean things and can't get away. I just want to get away from the stuff that makes me upset. I don't want to be a jerk, and most people like me, but they also wonder where I have gone a lot of times because I just like to leave. If people hurt my feelings, I just walk away and don't like to be around them again.

Checking for Understanding: *So, what do you think? Which animal sounds the most like you?* (Listen to and discuss their answers.) *Hmmm . . . I wonder when the last time is that you can remember acting like* (stated animal?) *That is a great example because you were feeling (afraid, unloved) you acted kind of like (Eddie, Contessa, Brutus, Sharla.) Great job!*

Individual (Brain-Changing) Practice: *Now, I would like to play a song about these characters. Let's listen to it one time and then do a puppet show the next time through the song where the animals act out the words!* Listen and then let the child get behind a table or chair to act out the puppets' song.

Session Summary: *Great job today, learning these characters, so remember I said I would see if you remember their names? I will hold them up, and you tell me their name and something about how they act.* (Allow the child to answer) *Sooo awesome!! I would like us to pay attention this week when we start to act like (Brutus, Contessa, Sharla, or Eddie.) I want to hear about it next week. Thanks so much! Let's put everything away except for the puppets, and I would like you to introduce them to your Mom and Dad. Let's go get Mom and Dad in the lobby!*

Fireballs of Pain

> **Restoration Therapy Steps One to Two**
> **Age Level: 5–16**
> **Materials needed: Five superballs and masking tape, markers**
> **Treatment Objective**: The child will learn how to identify and recognize painful emotions like pain and consequently want to respond by coping somehow. They will also begin to identify coping.

Buy in and Focus: *Tell me about a time when you have been in physical pain? Now tell me about a time when you have been in emotional pain?* (If prompting needed) *for instance, when did someone hurt your feelings, or when has something sad happened in your life?* (Listen to the child and empathetically reflect the story to them.) *What are some of the things you felt when this happened? What were some of the thoughts you had about yourself when that happened?* (try to dig to get to some of their painful core emotions and validate the pain.)

Psychoeducation: Explain that pain is pain. *Our brain recognizes physical and emotional pain in the same place, and we respond very quickly by going into fight or flight and acting out.*

Modeling (show): Without notifying the child, lightly toss a superball their way. Note their response to block, catch it, or what they did if it hit them unaware. Talk through what it felt like to have the superball come their way. Ask them to imagine if someone were to throw the superball at them as hard as they could, right at their nose. How would they maybe feel? What would they do? By first, observing and then hearing their response, it should provide some insight into their coping methods. Take note if their response is under the umbrella of blame, shame, control, or escape.

Intervention (practice alongside): Help the child construct labels to stick the child's painful feeling words onto three or four superballs. Use masking tape or a label maker to stick individual pain words on each separate ball. (Explaining to the child.) *These are kind of like fireballs. Let's pretend that they are like a little ball of fire, and they burn when they hit us. Okay, throw one at me!* (Yell ouch and maybe fall down. Then pick it up and yell ouch again as it touches your hand.) *Do you think I should pick it up? Should I put it in my pocket? Should I keep it in my hands and stare at it and carry it everywhere with me?* At this point, the child will likely be very animated and drawn in with problem-solving. *What are some things we might be able to do to protect ourselves from these balls of fire being thrown at us? They hurt!* (Allow the child to continue problem-solving.) *I agree. I think we need a shield because these words are painful. I think in one of our next sessions, we will make a truth shield. Yes, I think that will work well.*

Checking for Understanding: *So, tell me again what these balls represent or what these balls stand for. I wonder why we made and put labels on the balls. What do you think? Hmmm . . . yes, and they remind us that we all have painful feelings that sometimes hit us out of nowhere, and they hurt!!! It is good for us to know the names of the feelings we have that keep hurting us.*

Individual (Brain-Changing) Practice: *Tell me about another time when you were upset, when something happened that made you sad or mad or afraid.* (Allow the child time to answer and reflect his story to him to make sure there is a good understanding.) *When that happened, what were you hearing about yourself? What were the painful words that you heard about who you were? Oh, I see; yes, those are almost like the same words. Go ahead and write them down on the tape and let's stick these on the other Superballs. Are these words fierier than the others or less? The same?* This ranking gives us a good idea of which painful feelings are most painful.

Session Summary

Thank you for playing with the fireballs today. It helped me to understand better the painful feelings that sometimes hit you. I hope we can start to look at the painful feelings and then try to think of some calming words instead of reacting.

I am looking forward to coming up with some words that can put the balls of fire out. Does that sound good? Alright, let's pick up the toys and go and get Mom and Dad.

Take Care of Your Heart

Restoration Therapy Step Three
Age Level: 5+
Materials Needed: Teddy Bear named "Hardy."

Treatment Objective: The child will define and analyze the importance of taking care of their own heart first and foremost to have peace help others.

Buy in and Focus: Play the YouTube video "You Poked my Heart." Song. Then play "You Can Count on Me Like One Two Three" by Bruno Mars. *What do you think of this song? Do you think our friends or even parents will ALWAYS be there for us? NO MATTER WHAT?* (Allow for answer) *Well, we would like that, huh? But they can't be there all of the time. We do have some good friends or good family members, but even those good friends and people cannot be there all of the time, and they have bad days and might not be nice constantly, even if they are nice most of the time. What can we do if other people can't be there for us when we need someone to be gentle or kind or care for us when our hearts are hurting?*

Play the song "Be Kind to Yourself" by Andrew Peterson and discuss ways to be kind to ourselves. Point out that we are really the only ones who will always be around and who can always choose to take care of our hearts.

Psychoeducation: *When our emotions are hurting, it is very important, more than anything else, to keep our hearts safe and loved. What do you think I mean when I say, "Above all else, guard your heart because it is where life starts?"* (Proverbs 4:23) *Can you tell me what the heart does? Yes, it pumps blood into the rest of us, our arms, our brains, and our toes. If our hearts aren't working right, the rest of us won't work right either. So also, the heart talks about our emotions. It is where our emotions start too. When our emotional heart feels broken or hurt, the rest of us stops acting like it should. So, we need to protect it. It is a most important job! I wonder, what are some ways to protect our hearts?*

Modeling (Show): *So, let's pretend that this little teddy bear is named Hardy. What are some ways that his feelings may get hurt? Hmm . . . yes, that is a good one, or maybe if a kid at school says he is scrawny and weak, or his Dad is drinking or taking drugs, or if his parents get divorced or leave him.* (Add some of the child's specific painful experiences.) *Ahh . . . yes. Ouch, these things hurt!! When these things happen, it is almost like someone is punching Hardy in the face or slapping him, or poking him. Like this: "Hardy, you are dressed so ugly today. Why do you always look like such a nerd?"* Poke Hardy the Bear hard in the chest. *"Hardy, you can't do anything right!"*

Intervention (practice alongside): *Hardy is like our heart. Other people can say or do mean things that cause Hardy to hurt. He can start to feel very unsafe or unloved when things like these happen. He might feel like he needs to say what a bad kid he is, get BIG and ANGRY, run away and escape, or start to control things. But guess what? Do you think these things will help him? You are right; they will not! They will only end up hurting Hardy more. What is Hardy's number one job right now when he is hurting? His number one job is to take care of himself. How can he do this? Let me guess first . . . should he say something like, "I do dress so ugly, and I am a big nerd." Or maybe, "They are right; I can never do anything right. I am so stupid. My parents are probably getting divorced because I am such a dumb* *nerd."* At this point, the child will probably stop you.) *Yes, you are right! This is not a good way to take care of our hearts. So, let's talk about some things we can do that will take care of our hearts.*

Checking for Understanding: *So, I would like to ask you some questions. Is that okay? Who is Hardy? Yes, he is like our hearts that we need to take care of. What is our number one job when our hearts or feelings get hurt? Yes! Our number one job is to take care of our hearts. What are some things we might feel like doing when our heart is hurting that are not good for us? Yes, blame, shame, control, escape.*

Individual (Brain-Changing) Practice: Guide patients to identify their pain cycle and create an awareness that the pain cycle is "hurting their heart." *Okay, let's practice. Go ahead and pick up Hardy. What are some mean things people have said to your heart? Can you say them to Hardy? Oh wow. That is super sad and hurtful. Let me see Hardy.* Hug Hardy and perhaps kiss him on the head. *I am so sorry that those things happened to hurt you.* Begin to tell Hardy the child's suspected "truth" words. *Hardy, you are so lovable and smart and special.* Turn to the child and hand Hardy over to them. *Now I would like you to tell Hardy those same things or something that may even make him feel better.* Allow the child to practice. (Encourage the child to repeat it at least three times. You can also lead the child in a march around the room, down the hall, or in place repeating these "truth" words.

Session Summary: *Oh, my goodness! You did such a great job learning today about the most important thing we need to do when our feelings are hurting. To take care of our hearts so that the rest of us can work the way it needs to. This week, I would like you to practice noticing when your heart is hurting and the feeling. Then, instead of blaming, shaming, controlling, or escaping. Let's take care of hearts and tell it the things we told Hardy. Alright? Let's pick up the room and go get Mom and Dad.*

Empty Chair Bear

Restoration Therapy Step Two
Age Level: 5+
Materials Needed: Teddy Bear, Empty Chair
Treatment Objective: The child will externalize their emotional pain to learn to help regulate emotions and make healthy choices.

Buy in and Focus: *So today, we will bring a magic chair into the room. Does that sound okay? Okay, let's go get it.* Lead child to help you get a folding chair or extra chair. Bring it into the room. *Do you know any magic tricks?* Allow the child to show you their trick. *Oh, my goodness!* If they do not have a magic trick, feel free to use your favorite simple magic trick. There are many magic tricks available online. *So, we will do something kind of cool with this empty chair and a bear today. Does that sound okay?*

Psychoeducation: *So this Bear is named Empty Chair Bear. Can you say that five times fast? Great job! Since his name is sort of long, let's call him ECB. Okay, let's put him over here sitting in this big chair. Let me tell you a little bit about him and as I tell you about him, try to picture his story with me. I know his story will teach us some things about learning to take care of him and ourselves.*

Modeling: Come up with a story not exactly like the child's painful story but very close. *The following is an example. So . . . ECB is a good bear. He doesn't really like to get into fights with his little brother, but sometimes he gets really upset with his brother and even hits him. Then he feels bad, and he gets in BIG trouble, especially because his brother has autism. He doesn't really mind that he has autism, but sometimes, ECB's feelings get hurt because Mom and Dad pay A LOT more attention to his little brother than they pay to him. How do you think this might make ECB feel? Ah, yes, I agree he probably feels all alone, unimportant, and afraid. I wonder if you have ever felt like ECB before.* Allow for an answer and explanation.

Individual (Brain-Changing) Practice: Move into helping the child practice helping the Empty Chair Bear regulate his emotions. *You did a good job coming up with ideas to help ECB. So, tell me, what do you think ECB needs to hear from you so he can start to feel better?* Allow for answers. *I agree. Go ahead and look at ECB and tell him these things. Hmm . . . How is ECB feeling now? Oh, I am glad he is starting to feel better. What is something else that we can do for ECB to help him feel better?* Allow for answers. *Awesome! I agree, and do you think he may need a hug? You can hug him. What do you think ECB might need after getting back to his house tonight and seeing that his Mom and Dad are paying so much attention to his little brother again?* Allow for an answer; feel free to curiously add ideas if needed and ask if the child thinks your idea(s) would work or not? These answers will give you insight into what the child needs. *Those are really, really good ideas!*

Checking for Understanding: *I wonder if you can tell me how ECB was feeling when he first was sitting in the big chair? Yes, and then I think something magical happened, and he started to feel better? What helped him to feel better? I agree you thought about what he needed to hear, and you told him very kind and true things. I can see he looks more peaceful now and not so upset. Great job!*

Individual (Brain-Changing) Practice: *I wonder if ECB may feel some similar emotions to you? What sorts of things might make you feel better when you are upset? What things do you need to hear? Hmmm . . . I think those things are wonderful things to say to yourself when you are upset. Things like "I am important, I am lovable, I am a good enough kid!" This week, I would like you to practice saying these wonderful things when you start to feel terrible, like ECB before the magic of true words helped change him in that chair.*

Session Summary: *Today was so good. I liked how you helped ECB and told him true things about himself when he believed lies. I can't wait to hear how your practicing goes this week. Remind me, what are you going to practice this week? Awesome! Alright, let's put the chair and ECB back and go get Mom and Dad.*

Pete the Pain Eater

Restoration Therapy Step One
Age Level: 5–11
Materials Needed: Stuffed Toy with Zipper Mouth. (Purchased online) or a Puppet.
Treatment Objective: Help the child to identify painful feelings.

Buy in and Focus: Warmly invite the child into the session. Ask the child what was a high point of the week and what was a low point? While the child is talking through low points, listen to see if they identify any painful feelings. *I am glad to hear that you had some good times this week. Even when we are sad or hurt, it is important to remember that there are always good times. So today, I want you to meet a friend of mine. His name is Pete, and he likes to eat something strange. Are there any weird things that you like to eat?* You can add something weird you like to eat as well.

Psychoeducation: Grab "Pete the Pain Eater." *This is Pete. He likes to eat something very weird. Do you want to guess what it is? Those are good guesses; that would be weird! I think it is even stranger than that. He likes to eat painful feelings! What do you think about that? He gets really hungry for them, and it works out because it is helpful to us.* Lift Pete the Pain Eater up to your ear and pretend to listen, then nod. *Well, he is hungry and needs some painful feelings to eat. Let's help him.*

Modeling (show): *Here's what we will do. I am going to take this marker and tear off a piece of this paper. I am going to write a painful feeling on it like this.* Write down the word "alone." *Now, I will fold up this paper. Would you like to unzip Pete the Pain Eater's mouth and put it in there?* Allow the child to help and zip up the mouth again. If using a puppet, turn the puppet upside down and put the paper inside the puppet, saying *he likes his food to go straight to his stomach.*

Intervention (practice alongside): *Now, let's write our painful feelings on this paper as many as we can think of. I will let you write them, and then we will read it and tear the word off the paper and feed it to Pete, the Pain Eater.*

Checking for Understanding: *So, tell me what Pete likes to eat? What does he get hungry for? Very good! He eats painful feelings.*

Individual (Brain-Changing) Practice: Guide the patient to practice individually. If the child is very young, it may be difficult for them to write the words. If they can write even a little bit, be patient as they write the word. Spelling does not matter. Praise them for doing a good job writing the words. After the word is written, ask them to read it to you. Validate emotion compassionately. Ask them when they remembering feeling that way? Be patient to understand the and context and curiously and gently ask questions. After validating their pain, remind them that Pete the Pain Eater is hungry. Allow them to feed Pete and zip his mouth closed. Repeat this as many times as possible. Allow them to write all the painful feelings they can remember feeling. When they seem done, ask if there may be anymore.

As you are dealing with acute emotional pain, it is important to be nurturing, gentle, and compassionate throughout the exercise as your client relays hurtful experiences.

Session Summary: You did such a good job! Thank you for sharing your pain with both of us. Now it is really interesting and peculiar, but next time you come to visit. These painful feelings aren't going to in his stomach anymore. Pete likes to digest these things at night, so I think they will be gone next time you come. All eaten up! Make sure you remind me to check. Let's put him on the shelf and tidy up and then go get Mom and Dad!

Pain to Peace Flashcard Match-Up Game

Restoration Therapy Step One to Two
Age Level: 5+
Materials Needed: RT Pain and Peace Flash Cards, Four Steps Song
Treatment Objective: The client will identify, analyze, and comprehend their pain and peace cycles and how they feed into each other.

Buy in and Focus: Warmly welcome child into the session. Ask them how their week has gone. Ask them about what one of their favorite songs is. Then listen to the song together. (This is easily done as most popular songs are free to play online.) Ask what sorts of songs make the child feel sad and which kind of songs cause them to feel happy. After this discussion, play the RT "Pain to Peace" song to introduce the flashcard activity. Explain that this song will help us to learn the four steps to help us feel better, and so will the flashcards.

Psychoeducation: *I would like us to think about a time when we were in a conflict. Do you know what the word conflict means?* (allow the child time to answer.) *Thank you for trying to figure that out. Conflict means a disagreement or an argument. Can you tell me about a time you had a disagreement, like when you wanted to do something, and someone else wanted to do something else? Ahh . . . I like that example. Yes, so when we disagree or get in a fight or with people, it causes us to have painful feelings. Lenny, the Lying Lizard, lies and says we better act fast and become like one of the Coping Characters.* Show the child the puppets or pictures of Brutus the Blaming Badger, Sharla the Shame-Filled Sheep, Contessa the Controlling Cow, and Eddie the Escape Goat. *Remember these guys? Good, so the Pain to Peace Flash Cards will help us figure out what our four steps are. Then we can feel better, just like in the song.*

Modeling (show): Show the emotion flashcards, which are grouped in four different categories. The separate categories are labeled as Feelings, Coping, Truth, and Actions. *Now, we will choose the top three or four cards from the Feelings category first. We do this by thinking about when we are in a disagreement or conflict. Which feelings do we typically feel the most? Then we will pick the top three or four ways we cope and make a match with each particular feeling.*

Next, we will pick the top three or four cards from the Truth category, typically the opposite of the Feeling category's words. Lastly, we will choose the top three or for cards from the Action category, which describe how we usually act when listening to the Truth words. As you explain the process, arrange the cards on the floor or coffee table in a similar structure to the pain and peace cycle displayed on the handouts.

Intervention (practice alongside): Lead the client through the steps of the process, starting with asking the child to pick out their top three or four feelings that happen most often when they have a conflict or disagreement. Feel free to talk through each pick at length, asking what happened the last time that felt that particular feeling. Next, ask them how they typically react when they are feeling these emotions. Ask them to pick three or four cards from the coping pile. Next, point to the Feeling words they have chosen, and one by one, ask them to pick out an opposite card from the Truth category. Spend some time talking over the Truth words. Ask how they might remember these our true words? We can ask about family members or friends who agree with the Truth statements; we can incorporate faith to ask them about them working to believe this about themselves. We can let them know we firmly believe these things to be the truth about them. Lastly, we can read the Truth words slowly several times. While we do this, encourage the child to get comfortable and let the words soak in. Ask what this feels like. Then ask them to tell you, from this feeling of peace, how might we act differently. Allow them to choose three or four action words. Arrange them in the same format as the pain and peace self-perpetuating cycle. Point out that they feed into each other.

Checking for Understanding: You can now use a variety of strategies and questions to check for understanding. *Remind me what the word conflict means? When we are in a disagreement, what kind of feelings might we have? How can we help ourselves to feel better?*

Let's remember the four steps of the song:

1. Say what you feel
2. Say what you usually do
3. Tell myself the truth
4. Change actions

Now let's see if you can tell me what you usually feel in conflict? What things do you usually do? What is true? How might your actions change?

Individual (Brain-Changing) Practice: *You did an AMAZING job. We will continue to work on this together. I will take a picture of these cards and send it to your phone or make a photocopy for you to take home. When you start to feel pain or start to cope, let's start remembering these four steps.*

Session Summary: *Today, we learned a little more about discovering our pain and peace cycle and the four steps. Let's put the cards back and go grab your Mom and Dad.*

From Blaming to Boosting

Restoration Therapy Step: Skill Building and practice, after steps have been taught initially

Age Level: 5+

Materials Needed: Brutus the Blaming and Boosting Badger pictures, puppet and Coping Character Song and lyrics

Treatment Objective: The client will identify and practice how to move from the pain to the peace cycle, particularly from blaming to encouraging others

Buy in and Focus: Welcome the child into the room and bring the Badger puppet out placed on hand. *Do you remember this guy? What is his name? Correct, his name is Brutus the Blaming Badger.* Show the child the picture of Blaming Brutus. *Tell me more about Brutus. What is he like? Very good. Remember that whenever something happens that hurts Brutus's feelings, he usually tries to get very BIG and LOUD and points his finger at people and says, "This is your fault!!" I didn't do anything! He also calls people names and says stuff like, "you are so stupid." Let's listen to the Coping Character's Song again. This will help us to remember. Here are the lyrics so we can follow and sing along too!* Play the song and sing along with the client.

Psychoeducation: *When any of us experience conflicts or disagreements, we react like the coping characters because our hearts start feeling very sore and panicked. Can you think of a time you experienced feeling like this during a hard time?* Allow for an answer and validate emotion. *Yes, well, Brutus has had some hard things happen to him. When he was a badger cub, things were good; his parents and little sister were happy. They would take him down by the river to play, where his Dad taught him to dig for worms. "Look at little Brutus!" his Dad would proudly exclaim. "His paws are like shovels!" Because they were European Badgers, they happily shared their warm burrow with their forest family and friends. After some years, Brutus's grandma died. He had never felt so sad and alone. His grandma took care of him every day after school while his parents were at work. It was decided that Brandie the Rabbit would move in for a while to help around the burrow; badgers are very fussy about cleanliness. Brandie was very fancy, and she wore fake eyelashes, red lipstick, and smelled good. Brutus liked her but didn't like how his Dad started to spend so much time with her. His Mom did not like it either! She started to yell at his Dad a lot and would bare her teeth and click her claws together whenever Brandie's name came up. One night Brutus's Dad said he had had enough! He was sick of being a badgered husband! Brutus's parents told him that they were going to get a divorce. Dad was moving to another burrow with Brandie. Brutus immediately wondered if this was all his fault because Brandie had to move in to take care of him in the first place. His grandma left him, now his Dad and Brandie left him. He felt so unloved, rejected, and alone. When he started to have these painful feelings, he got really angry! When he got really angry, he yelled at his Mom and sister and bared* *his teeth. This seemed to make him feel better for a little while. But then guess what happened?* (Allow time for answers)

Well, his sister got scared to be around him, and she didn't want to play with him anymore. Also, his Mom said if he was going to act so angry, loudly, and hit his sister, that he couldn't live in their burrow, and he would need to go to Dad's. This made him feel more unloved, which fueled his anger. He was so mad he was being made to live with a fake Mom with fake eyelashes! Brutus was extremely upset with his Dad., so he started acting like a real jerk everywhere. He complained constantly, got into fights at school, and soon got suspended. Oh my! In the moments when things were quiet, he thought about how he didn't have many friends anymore, and no one seemed to want to have him around. Underneath everything, he just felt terrible! He did not want to be such a big jerk, but it was hard for him to feel like he could act differently because his heart was so sore. I wonder how Brutus could start feeling and acting better? (Allow the child time to answer.)

Modeling (show): *So, go ahead and grab one of the puppets. Let's act this story out together. Let's help Brutus make some different decisions instead of getting angry. I will be Brutus first, and you be a friend trying to help me.* Holding and speaking through Brutus the Badger puppet, speak very angrily and act hard to deal with. Use blaming words when interacting with another puppet. Model behavior for the child to feel comfortable engaging in free dialogue and puppet play.

Intervention (practice alongside): *So, I would like you to be Shalom, the Dove of Peace. Shalom is very important and loving, and safe. She can tell Brutus the truth about himself. Remember Brutus feels unloved, alone, and worthless. He is still acting mean, but she can remind him that he is not those terribly painful things that he is believing about himself.* Continue acting and speaking out Brutus's bullying behaviors while encouraging the child to use Shalom to speak the patient's truth words to Brutus. *It will be helpful for You to have Shalom repeat the Truth words to Brutus many times.* Using the Brutus puppet, ask Shalom to repeat the words. As the client repeats Shalom's words, take a deep breath.

Wow! I am starting to feel so much better. I usually feel very alone, and when I feel alone, I get angry and blame other people. But the truth is that I am not alone. I have friends. My grandpa loves me a lot, and he lets me call him anytime I want to. When I understand I am not alone, I want to act differently. I want to be Brutus the Boosting Badger!! I know that boosting other people up is the opposite of tearing them down; it is helpful, positive, and encouraging. Actually, now that I think about it, don't you think I will have more friends when I am a Booting Badger? Shalom, can you tell me what you think would be more helpful ways for me to act?

Checking for Understanding: *I think we did a great job with our puppet show. Can you remember why Brutus gets so angry and hits and acts in mean ways? Correct! Because his heart was very sore about his parent's divorce and he started to think it was his fault because he was not loveable, he felt alone and worthless, so he acted mean. What are the true things about Brutus? What did Shalom remind him of? Very good. She reminded him that he is loveable, not alone, and valuable when* *he started to think about these Truth words that happened. How did he want to act? Yes! He wanted to be a Boosting badger. What does boosting mean? Great job!*

Individual (Brain-Changing) Practice: *So, I wonder if we ever have felt like Brutus? Hmmm . . . yes and sometimes we can start acting very angrily and like a bully. What are some true things you can remind yourself of this week? Awesome! I want you to start practicing and practicing, reminding yourself of these true things!*

Session Summary: *You did a great job today helping Brutus go from Blaming to Boosting. I am excited to hear about your practicing next time we meet. Let's pick up the puppets and put everything away, and then go get Mom and Dad. You are such an important helper. You are a boosting kid right now!*

From Shame-Filled to Self-Assuring

Restoration Therapy Step: Skill Building and practice, after steps have been taught initially

Age Level: 4 to 11

Materials Needed: Sharla the shame-filled sheep pictures, puppet, and Coping Character song and lyrics

Treatment Objective: The child will identify and practice how to move from the pain to the peace cycle, particularly, being shame-filled to self-assuring

Buy in and Focus: Welcome the child into the room and bring the Sharla the Sheep puppet out on your hand. *Do you remember this sheep? What is her name? Correct, her name is Sharla the Shame-Filled Sheep.* Show the child the picture of Shame-Filled Sharla. *Tell me more about Sharla. What is she like? Very good. Remember that whenever something happens, that hurts Sharla's feelings, she usually tries to get very small and to disappear. She points the finger at herself and gets very self-conscious, and says, "This is all my fault!!" Why do I ever say anything at all? She calls herself a lot of mean names and thinks she is so stupid and dumb and doesn't look good to anyone." Let's listen to the Coping Character's Song again. This will help us to remember. Here are the lyrics so we can follow and sing along too!*

Psychoeducation: *When any of us experience conflicts or disagreements, we react like the coping characters because our hearts start feeling very sore and panicked. Can you think of a time you experienced feeling like this during a hard time?* (Allow for an answer and validate emotion.) *Yes, well, Sharla has had some hard things happen to her. She has had people that she thought should love her do very hurtful and embarrassing things to her. One time she shared a really embarrassing secret with her friend, and her friend told everyone about it! She was so embarrassed and just wanted to shrivel up into the tiniest little ball of wool. She was so scared that she was going to get in big trouble. It felt like everyone hated her. I wonder if you might be able to guess something about this secret she was hiding.* (Allow the child time to answer.) If the client says something about their own story of abuse, it may be good to adapt Sharla's story to be very similar to their own story but not exactly the same. *Thank you for sharing that idea with me of what Sharla's secret* *was. Well, Sharla told her friend that one day her Dad was watching the sheep-shearing contest, and he was rooting for his favorite farmer to win, but the farmer lost. Sharla asked why the farmer lost, and her Dad started to scream and scream at her. He said she was a stupid idiot, and she never obeyed, and that she should be in her room doing her homework instead of bothering him all of the time. She stepped toward him to tell him she was sorry and to hug him, but he slapped her face very, very hard and told her to get out of his sight! She didn't know what to do, and so she went to her room and thought about what a dumb sheep she was and agreed that what her Dad said was right. She was a stupid idiot. She didn't deserve to go out and eat dinner in the pretty green field with the better sheep. Instead, she decided she would eat some left-over moldy oats in the corner of the stable. This ended up making her already very sore tummy feel even worse. She wanted to ask her Mom to help her to feel better, but she didn't because she didn't deserve any help. She found a dark corner of the Sheep pen to curl up in and lay there shivering and worrying all night. She felt terrible! She wanted to eat some sweet green grass and jump around in the meadow with the other sheep, but she didn't know how she could because her tummy and heart were so sore. I wonder how Sharla the Shame-Filled Sheep could start feeling and acting better?* (Allow the child time to answer.)

Modeling (show): *So, go ahead and grab one of the puppets. Let's act this story out together and help Sharla make some different decisions instead of crying, separating herself from her friends and eating moldy oats. I will be Sharla first, and you be a friend trying to help me.* Speak through Sharla the puppet. Act very sad, sullen, and crying when being talked to. Allow Sharla to be hard to deal with. Use self-shaming words when interacting with another puppet. Model behavior for the child to feel comfortable engaging in free dialogue and puppet play.

Intervention (practice alongside): *Now, I would like you to be Shalom, the Dove of Peace. Shalom is very encouraging and loving, and safe. She can tell Sharla the truth about herself. Remember, Sharla feels unloved, stupid, and worthless. Sharla is still acting sad and shame-filled, but Shalom can come and remind her that she is not those terribly painful things that she is thinking about herself.* Continue Sharla's self-shaming behaviors while encouraging the child to use Shalom to speak the child's truth words to Sharla. Have Shalom repeat the Truth words to Sharla many times. (This is very helpful!) Speaking through Sharla, the puppet, ask Shalom to repeat the words.

Wow! I am starting to feel so much better. I usually feel very stupid and worthless, and when I believe that I am stupid and worthless, I get shameful and blame myself. But the truth is that I am not stupid. I am smart. My teacher told me that. I need to believe her. I know that I am smart too. I can make good decisions. Some people love me and want to hear what I have to say. My Dad was in a very bad mood, and that was not my fault! When I remember these true things, I want to act differently. I want to be Sharla, the Self-Assuring Sheep!! I know that assuring myself is the opposite of tearing myself down. I can encourage myself and be positive and remember what is good about me. Actually, now that I think about it, don't you think I will have more friends, fun and feel more loved when I am more confident? Shalom, can you tell me what you think would be more helpful ways for me to act?

Checking for Understanding: *I think we did a great job with our puppet show. Can you remember why Sharla gets so sad and shames herself and hides from other people? Correct! Because her heart was very sore about her Dad yelling at her and calling her names. She started to think it was her fault because she was not loveable. Maybe something was wrong with her? She felt stupid and worthless, so she acted depressed was too sad to play or do anything fun or helpful or good. What is the truth about Sharla? What did Shalom remind her of? Very good. Shalom reminded her that she is loveable, smart, and a good enough sheep! When she started to think about these Truth words, what happened? How did she want to act? Yes! She started to become a self-assuring sheep. What does self-assuring mean? Great job!*

Individual (Brain-Changing) Practice: *So, I wonder if we ever have felt like Sharla? Hmmm . . . yes and sometimes we can start acting very sad and depressed avoiding our friends or things that are healthy for us. What are some true things you can remind yourself of this week? Awesome! I want you to start practicing and practicing reminding yourself of these true things!*

Session Summary: *You did an amazing job today helping Sharla go from shaming herself to becoming self-assuring. I am excited to hear about your practicing next time we meet. Let's pick up the puppets and put everything away, and then go get Mom and Dad. You are such an important helper and wonderful kid!*

Controlling to Cooperating

Restoration Therapy Step: Skill Building and practice, after steps have been taught initially

Age Level: 4 to 11

Materials: Contessa the Controlling Cow pictures, puppet, and Coping Character Song and lyrics

Treatment Objective: The child will identify and practice how to move from the pain to the peace cycle, particularly controlling to cooperating behaviors.

Buy in and Focus: Welcome the child into the room and bring the Contessa the Controlling Cow puppet out on your hand. *Do you remember this cow? What is her name? Correct, her name is Contessa, the Controlling Cow.* Show the picture of Contessa. *Tell me more about Contessa. What is she like? Very good. Whenever something happens that hurts Contessa's feelings, she usually reacts by being very bossy and wants to do everything on her own because she feels like she can do it the best. She also likes to work hard to get a lot of awards and do things perfectly. She works hard to get straight A's in school and things like that. She says things like, "I am the best at making decisions, and people should listen to me. I can do things the right way, and I won't let myself down. Just let me take this project over!" She starts to believe she has better ideas than everyone else. Let's listen to the Coping Character's Song again. This will help us to remember a little more about her. Here are the lyrics so we can follow and sing along too!*

Psychoeducation: *When any of us experience conflict or disagreements, we react like the coping characters because our hearts start feeling very sore, scared, and panicked. Can you think of a time you felt like this during a hard time?* (Allow for an answer and validate emotion.) *Yes, well, Contessa has had some hard things happen to her. When Contessa was a little calf, her Mom packed her bags and left to go to another pasture far away to live. Her Dad left nearly every night because he was so sad. He would go to the town barn and drink way too much milk, which made him very sleepy and weird acting.*

Contessa was left home alone with her little brother and sister. It was scary late at night when they would hear coyotes howling. She would shake and shiver and felt like crying. But she learned to hide it because it would make her little brother and sister more frightened. She would create games to play together and then go out and gather water and fresh grass for them to eat. When her Dad finally came stumbling home after another night with the bulls at the barn. She would take care of him too. He got headaches, and she would have to quiet the children and make sure he was covered up with a blanket on cold nights. As long as she kept up with all of her chores and made good decisions, it seemed to help her pain go away. Inside and underneath her very put-together look, her heart was hurting. I wonder if you can tell me some of the things that Contessa may have felt? (Allow time to answer). *Those are some really good ideas, yes. She felt very unsafe, insecure, and like she could never be quite good enough. When she felt these things, she would start to get very bossy with her brothers and sisters, and made too many chore charts for them. She would get very angry when her siblings did not follow the chart exactly, and sometimes, she would scream at them. She also pushed herself very hard to keep the house perfectly clean and be the best show cow on the farm. She cared too much about how she looked. It was stressful! I wonder if you might have any ideas of how Contessa the Controlling Cow could relax and start feeling and acting better?* (Allow the child time to answer.)

Modeling (show): *So, go ahead and grab one of the puppets. Let's act this story out together and see if we can help Contessa make some different decisions instead of being so bossy, angry, and stressed out. I will be Contessa first, and you be a friend trying to help me.* Speak through Contessa the Cow puppet acting very bossy, angry, perfectionistic, and stressed. Allow her character to be fairly hard for the child to deal with. Uses controlling words and phrases when interacting with another puppet. *JUST LET ME DO IT, OR DO IT EXACTLY AS I SAY! I DO NOT NEED YOUR IDEAS OR YOUR HELP!"* Continue to model controlling behavior to help children experience how their coping may affect others. Also, this helps them to feel comfortable engaging in free dialogue and puppet play.

Intervention (practice alongside): *Now, I would like you to be Shalom, the Dove of Peace. Shalom is very encouraging and loving, and safe. She can tell Contessa the truth about herself. Remember, Contessa feels unsafe, insecure, and like she can never be or do enough. Contessa is acting bossy, perfectionistic, and controlling. Still, Shalom, can come and remind her that she is not those terribly painful things that she is thinking about herself.* Therapist, speaking through Contessa, continues her controlling behaviors while encouraging the child

to use Shalom to speak the child's truth words to Contessa. It will be helpful to have Shalom repeat the Truth words to Contessa many times. Using
Contessa the puppet, ask Shalom to repeat the words. Speaking through
Contessa, *Wow! I am starting to feel so much better. I usually feel very stupid and
worthless, and when I feel stupid and worthless, I get shameful and blame myself.
But the truth is that I am not unsafe all of the time. There are a lot of safe people
and places. I am safe right here and now. I am empowered to make safe choices. I am
secure with a lot of my friends and at school. I am good enough. I need to believe
these things. I am presently safe; I am presently secure; I am good enough! My Mom
did not leave because I wasn't a good enough calf. My Dad doesn't drink too much
milk because I am not good enough either. These things are not my fault. When
I remember these true things, I want to act differently. I want to be Contessa, the
cooperating cow. I know that cooperating with others and working hand in hand is
the opposite of being controlling. I do not have the only good ideas and will be open
to other people's ideas and help. It is stressful to make every decision and carry the
responsibility of everything alone. I can ask other people for help and encourage them.
I can be a good partner. Actually, now that I think about it, don't you think I will
have more friends and feel safer when I allow other people to help and share the load?
Shalom, can you tell me what you think would be more helpful ways for me to act?*
(Allow the child to answer.)

   Checking for Understanding: *I think we did a great job with our puppet
show. Can you remember why Contessa gets so bossy and perfectionistic? Correct!
Because her heart was very sore about her Mom leaving her and her Dad drinking
too much at the Barn. She started to think it was her fault because she was not doing
everything right. She thought if she acted good enough, maybe her Mom could come
back, and her Dad would stop drinking. She felt scared and not good enough, so
she acted controlling and wouldn't accept help from anyone or let anyone else have
an idea. This made other people feel frustrated around her. What are the true and
good things about Contessa? What did Shalom remind her of? Very good! Shalom,
reminded her that she is safe, secure, and a good enough sheep! When she started to
think about these Truth words, what happened? How did she want to act? Yes! She
started to become a cooperating cow. What does cooperating mean? Great job!*

   Individual (Brain-Changing) Practice: *So, I wonder if we ever have felt like
Contessa? Hmmm . . . yes and sometimes we can start acting very bossy and want to
be perfect and never make a mistake. We all make mistakes, and that is a stressful way
to behave. What are some true things you can remind yourself of this week? Awesome!
I want you to start practicing and practicing, reminding yourself of these true things!*

   Session Summary: *You did a great job today helping Contessa to stop acting
so controlling. She has become a cooperating cow! I am excited to hear about your
practicing next time we meet. Let's pick up the puppets and put everything away, and
then go get Mom and Dad. I hope you feel safe and secure here. You are a wonderful
kid!* (Often kids who struggle with controlling tendencies want to organize the toys,
or leave the office in a particular way. If this is the case, feel free skip the pick-up, asking them to leave the room unorganized. Let them know you want to arrange things

differently. (Reassure them that it will be fine.) This can prove challenging for some children, and can be a practice in cooperation.

From Escaping to Engaging

Restoration Therapy Step: Skill Building and practice, after steps have been taught initially

Age Level: 4 to 11

Materials: Eddie the Engaging Goat pictures, puppet, and Coping Character Song and lyrics

Treatment Objective: The child will identify and practice how to move from the pain to the peace cycle, particularly from escaping to engaging others

Buy in and Focus: Welcome the child into the room and bring the Goat puppet out on your hand. *Do you remember this guy? What is his name? Correct, his name is Eddie the Escape Goat. Show the child the picture of Eddie the Escape Goat. Tell me more about Eddie. What is he like? Very good. Remember that whenever something happens, that hurts Eddie's feelings, he usually tries to disappear as quickly as possible and says, "I don't want to fight. Please can't we just get along!" He wants to run away, and feels very stressed out when anyone is disagreeing. He wants people to like him. Let's listen to the Coping Character's Song again. This will help us to remember. Here are the lyrics so we can follow and sing along too!*

Psychoeducation: *When any of us experience conflicts or disagreements, we react like the coping characters because our hearts start feeling very sore and panicked. Can you think of a time you experienced this during a hard time?* (Allow for an answer and validate emotion.) *Yes, well, Eddie has had some hard things happen to him. Eddie's house was very loud! Eddie's Mom and Dad fought with each other, and they fought with his older sister. It seemed that all everyone liked to do is argue and butt heads. Eddie knew all the other goats wanted to solve every problem by squaring off and ramming into each other as hard as they could. Eddie did not like to butt heads one bit! All it did was give him a headache, he thought it must give them headaches too. He felt very scared when his family was arguing, and it hurt his ears! His sister was a teenager, and sometimes she would sneak out at night and go frolicking over the hills with teenage Billy Goats. When she got home, she and their parents would butt heads over her being out eating weeds all night. Mom and Dad insisted these were not good for her to eat and yelled at her for making "terrible choices." His sister butted right back and sometimes threw dishes on the ground and slammed her door. Eddie loved his family. He did not understand why everyone had to scream and butt heads so often. When people got angry, he would shake, and shiver. He hoped he would never get yelled at, so he tried to be very good and quiet. He wasn't good at arguing and felt like his throat got really tight when anyone was mean. Sometimes he tried to speak up, but felt like he was choking. He would just leave and find a quiet place to try and calm down.*

On the outside, the other goats had no idea he was so nervous. He tried to look very cool and wanted to go unnoticed. He also had a learning disability, and when he looked at letters or numbers to try and read them, they would sometimes look all scrambled up or upside down. Sometimes his friends made fun of him. He was embarrassed, but he acted cool and like it didn't matter. He wanted to not draw any attention to himself. Everyone thought he didn't really care about much and was just a really calm and peaceful dude. Sometimes, though he knew he hurt his close friend's feelings, they told him that they didn't like the way he seemed to ignore them. They said sometimes they wondered if he even liked them or gave a rip about them. Eddie was usually quiet when they told him these things. He didn't know what to do. Underneath everything, though, he just felt terrible! He did not want his friends to be sad or think he didn't care because he did. He just got so, so scared when they called him out for leaving during disagreements. He hated fighting more than anything. But it was hard for him to feel like he could act differently because his heart was so sore. I wonder how Eddie could start feeling and acting better? (Allow the child time to answer.)

Modeling (show): *So, go ahead and grab one of the puppets. Let's act this story out together and help Eddie make some better decisions instead of escaping, getting too quiet, or hiding. I will be Eddie first, and you be a friend trying to help me.* Speaking (or not speaking) act through Eddie the Goat puppet, run away when the other puppet talks to him and hide. At times do not respond to the conversation at all or make up an excuse to leave. Model behavior for the child to feel comfortable engaging in free dialogue and puppet play. Ask the child to have their puppet throw a ball at Eddie and have Eddie be unresponsive. Remark that it is very hard to have fun or play a game with someone if someone doesn't throw the ball back or respond, even if they are scared or shy.

Intervention (practice alongside): *Now, I would like you to be Shalom, the Dove of Peace. Shalom is very important and loving, and safe. She can tell Eddie the truth about himself. Remember, Eddie feels scared, unknown, and powerless. He is still avoiding, hiding and being shy. Shalom can remind him that he is not really those terribly painful and scary things that he is thinking about himself.* Continue Eddie's escaping behaviors while encouraging the child to use Shalom to speak the patient's truth words to Eddie. It will be helpful for You to have Shalom repeat the Truth words to Eddie many times. Using the puppet, ask Shalom to repeat the words.

Wow! I am starting to feel so much better. I usually feel very scared, powerless and unknown. When I feel scared, I usually run away. But the truth is that I am presently safe. I am not really in danger right now. When I feel powerless, I avoid people to feel safer, but I do have the power to speak up and make good choices about what I need to take care of my heart. Also, when I feel unknown, I feel shyer and shyer. I withdraw because I think I am not worth taking people's time to get to know me. When I understand the truth that people do want to know me, I want to act differently. When I understand I am presently safe, powerful, and known, I want to change into Eddie, the Engaging Goat!! I know that engaging with other people is the opposite of escaping from and avoiding others or activities. Actually, now that I think about it, don't you think I will have more friends and feel more confident when I am an Engaging Goat? Shalom, can you tell me what you think would be more helpful ways for me to act?

Checking for Understanding: *I think we did a great job with our puppet show. Can you remember why Eddie escapes and gets shy and quiet when his family and friends disagree with him? Correct! Because his heart was very sore about his family fighting all the time and it worried him. He started to believe he was unsafe and powerless to speak up about his thoughts. Because he didn't share much about himself, he felt unknown and like no one wanted to know him! What are the true things that we learned about Eddie? What did Shalom remind him of? She was very good; she reminded him that he is presently safe, powerful, and worthy of being known when he started to think about these Truth words, what happened? How did he want to act? Yes! He wanted to be Eddie the Engaging Goat! What does Engaging mean? Great job!*

Individual (Brain-Changing) Practice: *So, I wonder if we ever have felt like Eddie? Hmmm . . . yes and sometimes we can start acting very shy and hiding and not allowing people to know us. What are some true things you can remind yourself of this week? Awesome! I want you to start practicing and practicing reminding yourself of these true things!*

Session Summary: *You did a great job today helping Eddie go from Escaping to Engaging in his relationships. I am excited to hear about your practicing next time we meet. Let's pick up the puppets and put everything away, and then go get Mom and Dad. You are such an important helper. You are an engaging goat by helping me!*

Experiencing Pain to Peace in my Body

Restoration Therapy Steps Two to Three
Age Level: 4–18
Materials Needed: Blank 8x10 paper, markers, or crayons
Treatment Objectives: The child will begin to identify moving from pain to peace by drawing a body outline and putting their painful words on their body outline. Then construct an alternate body outline and put their peaceful words. The child will describe how the body feels and responds differently in both forms.

Buy in and Focus: Invite the child into the room warmly. Ask them how their week was and validate the experience. Ask them to describe a time when they felt happy and a time when they felt sad. Ask them to notice the different feelings in their bodies as they told both stories. Talk about how we may feel happy butterflies in our chest or a smile on our cheeks when we are happy. Discuss how our tummies or hearts may feel hollow or heavy when sad. Let them know we will draw something together that will help us see what happens in our body with different painful or peaceful words.

Psychoeducation: Isn't it so interesting that we feel emotions in our bodies. Did you know emotions cause our body to react? Emotions have energy. What is energy? Yes! It is a power source that transfers in one way or another. Energy causes things to happen. When we plug a lamp into an energy source the energy makes the lightbulb respond by creating light and heat. What does the energy of humor do? If you told me a funny joke, what might I do? Yes! I will laugh. Can you tell me a joke? (Allow child to tell a joke and respond by laughing.) When we laugh does our body stay still and quiet? No! We make a fun noise and we usually shake from the feeling of joy and surprise it brings. Our bodies respond and react to joy but also to other things. Have you ever tried really hard *not* to laugh when something funny happened? Tell me about it. (Allow child time to talk.) It is very hard to hold still and try not to laugh. I wonder if it is like this for other emotions? Today we are going to talk about how emotions affect our bodies.

Modeling (show): Draw a picture of an outline of a body on an 8x10 piece of paper; it should be fairly large, and the inside of the outline open enough to add words.

Intervention (practice alongside): Lead the child through drawing their body outline on two separate pieces of paper. On the top of one paper, write their name and the word "Pain" (e.g.) "Charlie's Pain." On the other paper, write "Charlie's Truth" at the top. Work together to write the pain words in the areas of the body where they feel them. For instance, "afraid" may be near the stomach or shoulders. The word "unwanted" may be near the heart. After discussing the pain words and how our body responds, move to the next paper and body outline, entitled "Charlie's (Child Name) Truth." Together look at the pain words and ask the child what words they would rather feel instead. Write these words in corresponding places on the body. Talk through the difference of feelings when they are experiencing the Truth words.

Checking for Understanding: Ask the child what this exercise was like for them. Ask them what things they learned about painful feelings and the truth.

Individual (Brain-Changing) Practice: Guide the child to put a star next to the top three painful feelings they feel and then put a star next to three corresponding truth words. Have the child say, "Sometimes I feel (pain word), but the truth is that I am (truth word.) For example, sometimes, I feel (unloved) but the truth is that I am a (loveable) kid! Have them practice going over their top three pain and truth words verbally several times.

Session Summary: *Amazing! You did some wonderful work today figuring out that pain visits all of our bodies, sometimes in different places, and it hurts. We also learned if we remind those painful feelings of the truth that our bodies can feel a lot of peace and calm. Let's go ahead and pick up our stuff and put the colors and extra paper away. I will save our body outlines so we can use them again. Let's go get Mom and Dad!*

Hula Hoop Jump from Pain to Peace

Restoration Therapy Steps Two to Three (After Steps are initially taught)
Age Level: 5–16
Materials Needed: Two Hula Hoops, Pain and Truth Body Outline from Child's file.
Treatment Objective: The child will practice moving from their unique pain cycle to their unique peace cycle.

Buy in and Focus: Welcome child warmly. Inquire about their week and ask them if they felt mostly in a painful hard place or mostly in a peaceful place. Ask them to recall a time when they experienced both. Discuss this together and encourage them by reminding them that they are doing a great job and learning how to experience more peace.

Psychoeducation: *Remember our body outline that we made with the painful words and the truthful words? I still have it, here. It was important for us to know what our feelings are and what the truth is.* (Refer back to their initial stories and talk through when they experienced the pain and truth words written on each body outline.) *So, let me ask you a question, is that okay? Great. So, imagine if someone just explained to us how to play basketball, but we never ever actually tried it or practiced it. Do you think we would be good players? I don't either! So, we need to start practicing at least two steps today. They will help us improve and remind us of the truth when we feel sad. There are actually four steps, but we will practice two today and fill in the other two in another session. Are you ready?*

Modeling (Show): *Place two hula hoops on the ground at least two feet apart from each other) Okay, now I am going to put the (Child's Name) "Charlie's Pain" paper just above the first hula hoop and "Charlie's Truth" paper just above the second hula hoop. When I jump in the "Pain" hula hoop, I will pick a word and look at where I feel the word in my body. I will then say the word while putting my hand on that part of my body. For example* (put your hand on your stomach and say) *"I feel afraid!" Now I will jump out of that pain hula hoop into the Truth hula hoop and do the same thing. I will pick the opposite word, the one I want to experience instead.* Put your arms in the air victoriously. *"I feel secure!"* Model this back and forth several times.

Intervention (practice alongside): After you lead the patient through the steps, invite the child into the activity. *Okay, do you want to try it with me?* Feel free to coach alongside until they get the hang of it. After several jumps back and forth, call for a time out to check for understanding.

Checking for Understanding: *It looks like you have it! I wonder what it feels like to be in the pain circle rather than the truth circle.* (Allow the child time to answer.) *So, what do you think we are doing this exercise for? Yes! So, we can practice, so we can get better at knowing when and where we feel a painful feeling and then remind ourselves of the Truth.*

Individual (Brain-Changing) Practice: Guide patient back to jumping and verbalizing painful feelings and truthful feelings. Feel free to join in. You can even point to the words and have the child find the truth word more quickly each time.

Session Summary: *Oh, my goodness! We did a really good job moving from Pain to Peace, and I think we got quicker as we practiced. This is even something we could do at home. We can certainly remember what to do when our body starts to feel painful feelings. Alright! Let's pick up our hula hoops and put them back, and hand me the paper so that I can keep them. Thanks so much! Let's go get Mom and Dad!*

The Truth Shield

Restoration Therapy Step Three
Age Level: 5 to 16
Materials Needed: several paper plates, scissors, and staples Superballs, tape.
Treatment Objective: The child will identify, analyze, and practice self-regulating truth words

Buy in and Focus: Begin the session by asking the child how his/her week has gone. Validate experience and any emotional pain. Remind the child of the "fireballs of pain" activity they previously participated in. Ask if those words are still what they have been feeling. Tape the words on the Superballs together. *Today we are going to make a Shield of Truth together.*

Psychoeducation: Refer back to the fireballs of pain words and the coping characters. Allow the child to identify the corresponding coping characters that best fit their desires to act out when the fireballs of pain come at them. Discuss how this type of coping ends up getting us in trouble and eventually feeling worse. Ask if they wish they could have a sort of shield that could protect them from the fireballs of pain. Talk through what words are opposite words to the words on the fireballs, or words that feel peaceful, write them down together. Explain that we will make shields with the Truth words that will help protect us from the fireballs of pain.

Modeling (show): Demonstrate how to make the shields with your client watching. Cut a two-inch strip out of the middle of the first plates. (This plate can be discarded after cutting the strip.) This strip will be used as the handle for the "shield." Staple this two-inch "handle" on the side of the second plate that is curved upward. This should now look like a shield with a handle.

Intervention (practice alongside): Lead the child through the process of making enough Shields of Truth to "counteract" the number of fireballs of pain. On the face of each shield, ask the child to write (feel free to help) one of their Truth words. They can decorate it however they wish or draw faces on the shield depicting the truth word. (e.g.). If their word is "safe," they can draw a peace-filled-looking face depicting the word.

Checking for Understanding: *How might these Truth Shields help protect you from the Pain Fireballs? Sometimes our feelings can lie to us, like Lenny the Lying Lizard. Do you remember all the lies he says to you all the time?* Listen for their response. *The Truth Shield helps us not to believe things that aren't true. When we listen to the Truth words instead of the Fireballs of Pain, we feel at peace. So, can you remember what the Truth Shields help with?*

Individual (Brain-Changing) Practice: Allow the child to take command of the Truth Shields. Take the Fireballs of Pain and call out the name of each Pain Fireball as you toss it in the child's direction. The child will need to pick up the corresponding Truth Shield to block it. As the child picks up each Truth Shield, encourage them to say the word out loud as they block the pain ball. As you pick up the pain ball and say, "*UNLOVED!*" toss it at the client. At the same time, the Child picks up the corresponding shield and says, "*IMPORTANT!*" Then block the fireball. Feel free to go back and forth for some time. This is good brain practice for the child. The novelty and physical activity will aid in keeping it in their memory.

Session Summary: Explain that there are two more minutes to continue to play the game. After two minutes, ask the child some questions. *Who do you think won? Was the Truth Shield effective? Practicing this will make it easier and easier for our brain to remember when the pain words come up. We can imagine having our Truth Shield words block the painful feelings. "You did a fantastic job today! I really enjoyed our time together. Let's pick up our scraps and throw them away. I will save our shields so we can keep practicing, and after we are done, we will go and get Mom and Dad."*

The Four Steps Song and Practice

Restoration Therapy Step: Review of all four steps
Age Level: 5–16
Materials Needed: RT Four Steps Song and Lyrics, puppets
Treatment Objective: The child will define, analyze, and practice the Four Steps of emotional regulation.

Buy in and Focus: Welcome the child warmly into the therapy room. *How was your week? I would like to hear about something good that happened and something hard that happened?* Allow the child to answer and validate emotion. *When the good thing was happening, I would guess you were probably in your peace cycle. What about when the difficult thing happened? What were some things that you started to feel during that time?* Allow the child to answer.

I want to help us to be able to remember, really easily, what the steps are for us to take when we start to have a hard time. I wonder if there are any songs you have memorized. Can you sing the song to me or tell me the words? WOW! That is impressive. I have whole songs memorized too. Songs are usually easy to remember! I would like to learn a song together today. Let's get some puppets and have them sing along with us, or they can lip-sync.

Psychoeducation: *We have talked about our painful feelings and when we feel worried about being unloved or unsafe. When we feel this way we start to act like the coping characters. We talked about how mostly we might act like (state particular coping characters that depict the child.) When we start to act like "Contessa the Controlling Cow." We need to tell ourselves the truth that we are "presently safe." After we remind ourselves of the Truth, we will Act differently. We can be Contessa the Cooperating Cow instead of Contessa the Controlling Cow.*

Modeling (Show): *Here is a copy of the song to look at the lyrics while we play it.* Pick up a puppet and hold the lyrics up, pretending the puppet is singing.

Intervention (practice alongside): Play the song, sing along, and do this as many times as possible while keeping the child engaged. Feel free to lip-sync, use puppets, do a show, act it out, march around the room, dance. It is also fun to come up with some intentional choreography with the child to reflect the words of the song. The goal is to help the child memorize the four steps to access them when needed.

Checking for Understanding: *Great job singing the song! I feel like we are getting to know it pretty well. Can you tell me the four steps? Very good!*

1. Say what you feel
2. Say what you used to do
3. Tell myself the truth
4. Change my actions

Individual (Brain-Changing) Practice: *Alright, I would like to hear you sing the song by yourself or do a puppet show for me. Want to get Mom and Dad and show them the song?*

Session Summary: *You did a great job today starting to learn the song. I can't wait to see if you remember it next time we meet.*

Four Steps Song

by Micah John Frigaard

Step 1,2,3 4
when my heart is sore
I know the way
to help me feel better

Step 1 I say what I feel down in my heart,
Then say what I used to do, yeah that's the 2nd part
Then 3 sets me free; I tell myself the truth.
Then step 4 comes simply, change my actions. There's your proof

The proof to changing your pain to peace these are the easy steps that you can achieve

Step 1,2,3 4
when my heart is sore
I know the way
to make me feel better

Step 1,2,3 4
when my heart is sore
I know the way
to make me feel better
make me feel better better

Reference

Frigaard, M. (2019). *Pain to peace song*.

Index

Page numbers in *italics* indicate a figure on the corresponding page.

For Product Safety Concerns and Information please contact our EU
representative GPSR@taylorandfrancis.com
Taylor & Francis Verlag GmbH, Kaufingerstraße 24, 80331 München, Germany

www.ingramcontent.com/pod-product-compliance
Lightning Source LLC
Chambersburg PA
CBHW050613280326
41932CB00016B/3028